Praise for *How to Talk with Your Doctor*

This important and groundbreaking book bridges the great divide between traditional and alternative medicine. As Dr. Hoffman so astutely points out (and blends seamlessly in his own practice), the two can co-exist. It is time to forge this alliance for the optimal holistic approach to health, longevity and well-being—and this book provides the practical tools we need to make this happen. A must read for patients and physicians alike. Highly recommended!

—NICHOLAS PERRICONE, M.D., ADJUNCT PROFESSOR OF MEDICINE
AT MICHIGAN STATE UNIVERSITY 'S COLLEGE OF HUMAN MEDICINE, AND
FORMER ASSISTANT CLINICAL PROFESSOR OF DERMATOLOGY AT YALE SCHOOL OF
MEDICINE; BEST-SELLING AUTHOR OF *THE PERRICONE WEIGHT LOSS DIET,*
THE PERRICONE PRESCRIPTION, AND *THE PERRICONE PROMISE*

How to Talk with Your Doctor should be required reading for anyone who is frustrated with modern medicine—patients and physicians alike. In this engaging and articulate book, Ronald Hoffman, M.D., a pioneer in alternative medicine (with impeccable mainstream credentials, too), shows readers how to take charge of their healthcare and offers practical solutions for common health concerns. He also lays the groundwork for a new model of medicine that just might be the answer for our ailing healthcare system.

—JULIAN WHITAKER, M.D., FOUNDER AND DIRECTOR OF THE WHITAKER WELLNESS
INSTITUTE; AUTHOR OF *THE WHITAKER WELLNESS WEIGHT LOSS PROGRAM,*
DR. WHITAKER'S GUIDE TO NATURAL HEALING, REVERSING DIABETES, AND
HEALTH & HEALING, THE NATION'S LEADING HEALTH NEWSLETTER

How to Talk with Your Doctor serves as the long-awaited link between mainstream and complementary approaches to challenging medical issues as well as maintaining optimal health. Dr. Hoffman expands our vistas, allowing the reader to embrace the most comprehensive view of health and disease.

—DAVID PERLMUTTER, M.D., F.A.C.N., DIRECTOR OF THE PERLMUTTER HEALTH
CENTER AND PERLMUTTER HYPERBARIC CENTER; AUTHOR OF *BUILD A BETTER BRAIN*
BY KINDERGARTEN, THE BETTER BRAIN BOOK, BRAINRECOVERY.COM, AND *LIFEGUIDE*

Although the author points out that many practitioners of conventional medicine still express "outright scorn" for complementary and alternative medicine, times are changing. Medical schools across the land have physicians on their faculty who incorporate alternative therapies into both their practice and teaching. And today's medical students do indeed want to learn more about complementary medicine for the benefit of their future patients and themselves. It's quite a different environment from the one Dr. Hoffman found when he attended medical school. His book should help change this environment even further. The large amount of well-organized and well-written information about complementary and alternative medicine should be enormously useful to medical school professors and students alike.

—ALBERT S. KUPERMAN, PH.D., ASSOCIATE DEAN FOR EDUCATIONAL AFFAIRS
AT ALBERT EINSTEIN COLLEGE OF MEDICINE

Imagine melding the best of the conventional and alternative medicine worlds? This book offers practical hints and solutions to make this happen, by improving that seemingly simple, yet quite profound, time-honored essence of the sacred communication between patient and physician.

—KENNETH BOCK, M.D., PRESIDENT OF THE AMERICAN COLLEGE
FOR THE ADVANCEMENT IN MEDICINE; COFOUNDER AND CODIRECTOR OF
THE RHINEBECK HEALTH CENTER AND THE CENTER FOR PROGRESSIVE MEDICINE;
COAUTHOR OF THE GERM SURVIVAL GUIDE, NATURAL RELIEF FOR
YOUR CHILD'S ASTHMA, AND THE ROAD TO IMMUNITY

As one of the pioneers and leaders in complementary and integrative care, Dr. Hoffman provides us with an insightful guide for getting the best care in today's increasingly complicated and confusing medical system.

—JASON THEODOSAKIS, M.D., FORMER DIRECTOR AND CLINICAL ASSISTANT
PROFESSOR OF THE PREVENTIVE MEDICINE RESIDENCY TRAINING PROGRAM AT
THE UNIVERSITY OF ARIZONA COLLEGE OF MEDICINE; BEST-SELLING AUTHOR
OF THE ARTHRITIS CURE AND MAXIMIZING THE ARTHRITIS CURE

HOW TO TALK WITH YOUR DOCTOR

The Guide for Patients and Their Physicians Who Want to Reconcile and Use the Best of Conventional and Alternative Medicine

RONALD L. HOFFMAN, M.D., WITH SIDNEY STEVENS

Basic Health

PUBLICATIONS, INC.

The information contained in this book is based upon the research and personal and professional experiences of the authors. It is not intended as a substitute for consulting with your physician or other healthcare provider. Any attempt to diagnose and treat an illness should be done under the direction of a healthcare professional.

The publisher does not advocate the use of any particular healthcare protocol but believes the information in this book should be available to the public. The publisher and authors are not responsible for any adverse effects or consequences resulting from the use of the suggestions, preparations, or procedures discussed in this book. Should the reader have any questions concerning the appropriateness of any procedures or preparation mentioned, the authors and the publisher strongly suggest consulting a professional healthcare advisor.

Basic Health Publications, Inc.
28812 Top of the World Drive
Laguna Beach, CA 92651
949-715-7327 • www.basichealthpub.com

Library of Congress Cataloging-in-Publication Data
Hoffman, Ronald L.
    How to talk with your doctor : the guide for patients and their physicians who want to reconcile and use the best of conventional and alternative medicine / Ronald L. Hoffman, with Sidney Stevens.
        p. cm.
    Includes bibliographical references and index.
    ISBN-13: 978-1-59120-112-0
    ISBN-10: 1-59120-112-8
    1. Physician and patient. 2. Communication in medicine. 3. Integrative medicine. I. Stevens, Sidney. II. Title.

    R727.3.H579   2006
    610.69'6—dc22

                                                                    2006016608

In-house Editor: Cheryl Hirsch
Typesetting and Book design: Gary A. Rosenberg
Cover Design: Mike Stromberg

Printed in the United States of America

10   9   8   7   6   5   4   3   2   1

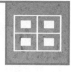

Contents

To my mother, Lina Hoffman,
1925–2005,
whose final words to me were
"Do the best you can."

Acknowledgments

I would like to acknowledge the following people and their unique contributions to this book:

Norman Goldfind, my publisher, who nurtured the idea for this book, and who has been a courageous longtime supporter of innovative medical concepts, even long ago at a time when complementary and alternative medicine was considered practically heretical and subversive. This book should serve as a vindication of his progressive views.

Jack Challem, an erudite health writer and researcher, whose inspiration gave life to *How to Talk with Your Doctor.* I am proud that by dint of writing this book I have been brought into closer association with an individual whose work I have long admired.

Sidney Stevens, who was indispensable to writing this book. Acting as advisor, facilitator, and sounding board, she played the role of enlightened healthcare consumer, patiently helping to clarify my ideas. She was the ideal collaborator, and made the sometimes lonely and grueling process of writing a book fun.

Laurie Cowan, my boon companion, who shares with me the vision of promulgating information that helps people and is indispensable to its realization.

The patients of the Hoffman Center, who for over twenty years have provided me with a living laboratory for applying the concepts in this book.

My dedicated staff at the Hoffman Center, who have supported my efforts to take on extracurricular projects like this book.

Radio listeners of "Health Talk," whose calls, letters, and e-mails have formed the basis for some of the examples in this book.

My wonderful friends and family, who have supported this project with encouragement and love.

My mentors and colleagues in the field of complementary and alternative medicine, too many to enumerate, whose teachings, personal courage, and collegiality have been an inspiration to me as I practice.

And lastly, to generations of doctors to come, who will face the challenges of integrating high-tech medicine and alternative treatments, and to twenty-first-century patients who are striving to reconcile the advice of health professionals with the latest breakthroughs in complementary and alternative medicine.

Preface

My journey into holistic medicine has been a rewarding trek, though not without its share of twists and detours. Along the way, I've discovered a whole new world of medical possibilities, but I've also confronted a few obstacles, too. In fact, that's why I'm writing this book. The obstacles—including outright scorn for the complementary and alternative approaches I embrace along with mainstream approaches—are some of the same obstacles that patients and their doctors continue to face as they set about merging the best of conventional and alternative medicine. By recounting my journey here and in the following chapters, I hope to share some of my insights and strategies with fellow travelers. My goal is to help both patients and doctors find the most effective therapies medicine has to offer, as well as foster more nurturing and collaborative relationships between them.

Where the Journey Began

My foray into alternative and complementary medicine really began in childhood. I was a science "geek" in grammar school. One of my first memories was the launch of Russia's Sputnik satellite on my fifth birthday, an event that set American schools scrambling to boost science literacy and catch up with the Soviets. I went above and beyond the call of duty; when a science report called for five pages, I turned in thirty—and that was fourth grade! I remember dissecting earthworms on my own, and my mother indulged my icky predilections by bringing beef eyeballs and hearts back from the butcher. By age fourteen, I was doing calculus in a college placement program for high school students at the University of California–Los Angeles (UCLA).

I did a "180" in college, though, virtually turning my back on the sciences. I reconfigured myself as a cross between Jack Kerouac and Alan Ginsburg, two "beat" writers who preached the virtues of bohemian rebellion. I even enrolled in their alma mater, Columbia University in New York. It was the early 1970s, a time of social and political foment, when pursuing conventional careers like medicine, law, and finance seemed "square" on hip Ivy League campuses. Instead, I

plunged myself into the humanities, devouring foreign languages, studying religion, history, and art; availing myself of the vast resources of New York City; and
even traveling to Europe, North Africa, and Israel to immerse myself in different
cultures.

When it came time to declare a major, the logical choice was anthropology.
Yes, it held an echo of science—digging up ancient remains and carbon-dating
them, studying the diets of remote tribes, even evaluating the sometimes bizarre
healing rites of shamans. But what really appealed to me was "anthro's" notion of
cultural relativism—the setting aside preconceptions about "superior" Western cultures and squatting with the natives for a while to see the world as they do. From
there, even the most "ridiculous" customs are seen as a culture's unique way of
dealing with the world—an approach every bit as sophisticated as our own, just
different. I didn't know it then, but this training would prove invaluable later as I
began navigating two seemingly incompatible medical worlds (conventional and
alternative), trying to blend the most effective healing approaches from each.

After college, I cut my hair and got a job with the City of New York. I enjoyed donning a suit every day and getting a paycheck, but still didn't know what
my life's work would be. As the clamor of the 1960s and 1970s gave way to a more
introspective time, I began drawing inspiration from the Far East. I meditated,
dined on vegetarian macrobiotic meals, and began studying acupuncture, yoga,
shiatsu, and herbal medicine. Gradually, I came to believe that much of value had
been lost in the West by abandoning older traditions.

"They're Not Looking for *Oddballs* in Medical School"

It was then that I hit upon the idea of going to medical school. It would be hard
after a four-year hiatus from college and minimal science training. But I was determined to become a holistic physician and began fast-tracking the training I needed.

After a two-year science refresher program, which included the *single* most
miserable summer of my life (*two* semesters of pre-med organic chemistry compressed into a frenetic twelve weeks), I was ready to submit medical school applications. In an accompanying essay I excitedly described how I hoped to legitimize
my interest in nutrition, natural remedies, yoga, and acupuncture with a firm
grounding in medical science. I was about to send in the applications, when an
older friend suggested I first run the essay by some doctors she knew for feedback.

I remember visiting one of them, fully expecting her to commend me on my
prose and my special "holistic" calling. But as she read it, her brow furrowed.

"Look," she finally exclaimed, "they're not looking for *oddballs* in medical
school!"

My heart sank.

"Go ahead and say that diet and exercise are important," she added. "Say that you jog and eat low-fat. They like that. But don't lay it on so thick about wanting to revamp the entire field of medicine. That stuff is *threatening*. Keep those cards close to your chest, kiddo, or else—*you ain't gettin' in!*"

I was discouraged and angry, but after showing the essay to other trusted confidantes, they pretty much agreed: "Don't give 'em more rope than they need to hang you!"

So I toned down the essay, and resolved to be the perfect "stealth" medical student, studious by day, while quietly pursuing my "holistic" interests after hours. Once I got into Albert Einstein Medical School, I pretty much stuck to the script—except for a few low-key side trips into alternative medicine. I started a nutrition study group, for instance, and served veggie alternatives, like "Tofu Pups" and soyburgers, at the graduation barbeque. I even took a couple of electives in acupuncture, medical hypnosis, and nutrition, and had a part-time job as a vegetarian cooking instructor. But otherwise, I was a model student, seldom proselytizing and rarely wearing my "holistic" colors on my sleeve. Mostly, I lay low observing like an anthropologist the often-bizarre rites of conventional medicine, which I studied tirelessly and mastered.

When it came time to apply for my residency, I did let my guard down once. My faculty advisor was a veteran internist, a blood-and-guts traditionalist who'd never left academic medicine for the "less pure" world of private, community-based practice.

During one visit he asked me which subspecialty among the many "-ologies," such as gastroenterology, endocrinology, and cardiology, captured my interest. When I answered honestly that I hoped to specialize in nutrition, he looked incredulous. "You mean you'd simply sit there and listen to patients, then proceed to tell them what to eat?"

"Well, yes," I said, "but there's a little more to it than that . . ."

I fully expected an angry outburst, but after an uncomfortable silence he finally sighed: "If you see patients that way you'll probably never make more money than a *psychiatrist!*"

So *that* was it! A gifted student in internal medicine squandering it all to offer mere talk therapy. Maybe he had a point . . .

A Few Steps Closer

It's twenty years later, and my decision to pursue a career in complementary and alternative medicine (CAM) has weathered the test of time. The very medical school where I was a "stealth" student now regularly invites me back to lecture to alumni and teach medical students. The federal government has recognized the legitimacy of CAM with multimillion-dollar research grants to evaluate its effectiveness. And I've become a recognized authority to patients and radio listeners alike.

But, even with this tremendous progress, medicine still has a ways to go. Many doctors continue to resist the idea of using CAM therapies, and a majority of patients still fail to bring them up, even when they're using alternative approaches on their own. What's more, many patients don't even receive the best conventional care, because they either fail to ask the right questions or because their doctor lacks the time to keep up with the latest medical thinking.

The result? Miscommunication and missed opportunities. Doctors feel increasingly burnt out and disillusioned, locked in a battle with demanding patients for control of their medical care. They may crave better relationships with patients, but don't always know how to make them happen. Nor are they convinced that listening and "talk therapy" are really the best uses of their time.

Patients, on the other hand, see their physicians as increasingly rushed, impatient, and set in "conventional" ways. They want to ask questions, expect answers, and trust that they'll be full partners in exploring *all* medical options. They're seeking an emotional bond, and their expectations are high. Yet as I discovered with my faculty advisor, too often they run up against a wall of resistance and lack of understanding. In the end, they fail to get the nurturing, attention, and respect they desire.

This book is for patients and doctors alike. My hope is to arm patients with the tools and knowledge they need to communicate better with physicians about using the best high-tech and alternative treatments, while also helping doctors balance their skepticism of CAM approaches with open-mindedness. The real goal is to foster a sense of mutual respect and open dialogue between doctors and patients that allows for the best care and most rewarding relationships possible.

In Part One, we'll look at how doctors are trained, what practicing medicine is really like, and why so many physicians still resist non-conventional approaches. We'll also look at how growing interest in alternative treatments is changing the practice of medicine and how it might change even further—for the better.

Part Two offers a blueprint for maintaining optimal health and dealing with chronic illness. It also explores complementary and conventional options for preventing and treating specific conditions, such heart disease, cancer, arthritis, and cognitive disorders like Alzheimer's disease. Separate Resource sections for patients and doctors offer products, websites, and organizations that can help promote more dialogue and medical collaboration.

Throughout my journey, I've seen profound changes in medicine that continue to this day. My long-held belief that medicine can—and should—be a fusion of alternative and high-tech approaches is now a reality in many places and continues to spread. The future is likely to bring a further merging of medicine's two worlds, as well as more satisfying partnerships between doctors and patients. My hope is that this book moves us all a few steps closer.

PART ONE

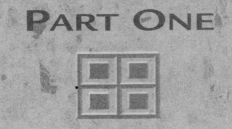

What's Wrong—
and Right—
With Medicine

Why Doctors Act the Way They Do

You will observe with concern how long a useful truth may be known
and exist, before it is generally received and practiced on.

—BEN FRANKLIN

It just keeps happening. I hear the same lines every day from patients. After checking with their conventional doctors about using natural or innovative therapies, they're given some haughty rebuff:

- "If this were so effective, every doctor in the country would use it."

- "The people who push these therapies have no scientific evidence to back them up."

- "You can't expect to find something that really works on the shelf of a health-food store."

- "What makes you think you're more qualified than me to make judgments about your medical care?"

- "These are nothing but rip-offs and scams!"

And yet, during my twenty-year medical career, I've been right, often as not, in championing cutting-edge therapies that were initially scorned. These include the following now well-accepted approaches:

- Going beyond cholesterol to predict cardiovascular disease risk with tests like HDL (high-density lipoprotein) cholesterol, homocysteine, C-reactive protein, lipoprotein (a), and the EBT (electron beam tomography) heart scan.

- Using glucosamine sulfate and chondroitin to treat arthritis.

- Treating ulcers as an infection.

- Using fish oil for a variety of disorders, from depression to colitis to cardio-vascular disease.

• Recognizing the benefits of a low-carbohydrate diet in battling America's epidemics of obesity and arteriosclerosis.

• Harnessing antioxidant-rich polyphenols from fruits, vegetables, tea, and spices to ward off arthritis, Alzheimer's disease, cancer, and heart disease.

• Preventing and reversing prostate problems with saw palmetto.

• Combating eye disorders, like macular degeneration, with antioxidant vitamins, minerals, and lutein.

These are just a few of the medical approaches that might have "died on the vine," if not for the determination of progressive researchers and clinicians. I'll provide more details on these revolutionary breakthroughs in later chapters. But for now they serve to illustrate how doctors themselves often overlook or block new, scientifically validated complementary and alternative approaches not to mention a few mainstream treatments as well. What's more, many physicians often fail to communicate their reasons for doing so, leaving patients frustrated, confused, and lacking in optimum care. Granted things are beginning to change as more mainstream doctors become curious about complementary and alternative medicine (CAM) and make an effort to learn what they can and reach out to patients. The next two chapters will examine these trends in more detail. However, many physicians still have a ways to go. This chapter will take a look at why that's so.

MEDICAL HERESY

Many people believe that medicine is a pure science, free from the taint of ideology or the marketplace. They're often surprised to find that it's actually fraught with tremendous bias against certain therapies. Take vitamin supplements, for example. Even with millions of users, conventional doctors still balk at recommending them. One reason is that vitamin advocates often operate outside the narrow scientific club (the "in" group) that defines what's medically acceptable. Nor has mainstream medicine fully embraced the notion of "deficiency diseases"—conditions like heart disease and cancer that may be preventable with the right vitamins and nutrients. Such thinking conflicts with the "find-a-bug, use-a-drug" approach that fuels so much pharmaceutical innovation and boosts drug company profits.

According to a recent article in the *Archives of Internal Medicine,* this irrational resistance may be similar to the church's indignation over Galileo's assertion that the Earth revolves around the Sun.[1] Simply put, supplemental nutrients and other CAM therapies defy conventional medical wisdom and threaten established thinking. "There are only three important questions when evaluating a potential treatment," the article concludes: "Does it work? What are the adverse effects? How much does it cost?" How it was developed and who advocates it isn't really relevant.

Unfortunately, just as Galileo was punished for his beliefs, modern medicine has maligned supplements by ignoring evidence that they work and by latching on to occasional bad news about their toxic effects. What's more, many physicians caution patients against vitamins, minerals, herbs, and other CAM therapies because they fear adverse interactions between them and conventional drugs. (Chapters on individual health conditions in Part Two explore disease-specific, drug–nutrient interactions in more detail, including common misconceptions and ways to learn more.) With so much negativity and fear surrounding the use of supplements and other CAM treatments, even doctors who personally believe in their effectiveness often find themselves hard-pressed to challenge mainstream medical thinking and recommend them to patients.

Supermarket Medicine

Most of us assume when we go to a doctor or hospital that we're benefiting from the latest medical innovations. But this is far from true. I call this "Supermarket Medicine."

Just as the market often dictates which foods make it to store shelves, it also decides what care patients receive. In the case of food, the latest, best, or safest products often never reach supermarket aisles because of inefficiency, lagging acceptance, lack of convenience, or sheer cost considerations. In most areas of the country "health food" is relegated to a few specialty stores.

Likewise, medicine is also subject to mass-market quirks and customs. Whether or not you receive a cutting-edge treatment touted in the latest medical journals, or even basic preventive care like diet and exercise advice, depends on who your doctor is, whether he or she keeps up with the latest advances, what your insurance company is willing to pay for, whether your doctor is afraid of being sued, how well a hospital is equipped, and even what therapies are in vogue in your local community.

"Ask Your Doctor About . . ."

For similar reasons, most patients also never hear about anything but dominant brand-name drugs from their physicians. They're told in direct-to-consumer ads to "Ask your doctor about . . ." And physicians—prodded by powerful drug companies to prescribe the pill *du jour* and pressured by health insurers to keep patients happy—have little recourse but to oblige. In fact, evidence suggests that many are as swayed by these ads as their patients.

Indeed, few mainstream doctors even know about alternative offerings from smaller companies simply because most can't compete with the pharmaceutical "big boys." Television and magazine ad pitches require financial resources only huge multinational drug companies can afford. "Guerilla-marketing" efforts by small, natural supplement businesses tend to pale by comparison, their products mostly languishing below the radar of mainstream medicine. Bottom-line: It's often the savvy patients who first learn about alternative products and either pass along the information to their doctors or simply use the products quietly on their own.

". . . But It's Not in the Scientific Literature!"

Harried physicians often struggle just to eke out enough time to translate mainstream medical research into drug prescriptions and new surgical procedures (see "A Day in the Life" on page 12). Indeed, many physicians learn about the latest medical breakthroughs the same way their patients do—while reading their morning papers or watching the news! So it's not surprising that even those few doctors who aren't biased against complementary or nutritional therapies often have no idea that thousands of pertinent CAM articles appear in the scientific literature each year.

Here are just a few examples:

• *Nutritional Therapy in Medical Practice* (2003 edition), a reference manual and study guide for physicians, by Alan Gaby, M.D. and Jonathan Wright, M.D., contains nearly 3,900 references from well-respected, peer-reviewed medical journals.[2]

• Numerous highly regarded medical journals (not health-food store magazines) are now devoted entirely to scientific investigation of alternative medicine and nutrition, including the *Journal of Alternative and Complementary Medicine, Alternative Medicine Review,* and the *American Journal of Clinical Nutrition.*

• A single Internet search on "Vitamin E and Heart Disease," for example, yields 11,599 "hits" from scientific journal references for the twelve-year period from 1991 to 2003.

• Fourteen separate, fully accredited conferences for doctors on complementary, integrative, and alternative medicine topics are listed on one quarterly calendar of medical events in the journal *Alternative Therapies in Health and Medicine* for February to June 2004.

• Even the ultra-orthodox *Journal of the American Medical Association* (JAMA) has joined in. In 2002 the journal published a landmark article entitled, "Vita-

mins for Chronic Disease Prevention in Adults: A Scientific Review," presenting thirty-five years of research showing that multivitamin supplements can
help lower the risk of certain chronic diseases in adults.[3]

It's not that "there aren't any studies," as many doctors claim. It's more a matter of awareness and acceptance. Many doctors simply don't know about the
abundant CAM resources available to them. And others choose to look the other
way. The result—continued resistance to integrative medicine. As renowned
Nobel Prize winner and vitamin C advocate Dr. Linus Pauling once noted, "If a
doctor's not up on something, he's likely to be down on it."

WHY DON'T THEY TEACH THIS STUFF
IN MEDICAL SCHOOL?

Twenty-five years ago when I entered medical school, complementary medicine
was just hitting the mainstream. Acupuncture and yoga were newly popular, and
Dr. Nathan Pritikin was making waves with his low-fat diet. I was fortunate to
be able to attend Albert Einstein Medical School, which was very open to new
ideas. The administration gave a group of us a few hundred dollars to start a
nutrition study group, where we eagerly sampled tofu while debating the benefits of the then hot-health trends like vegetarianism. I even managed to get one
of my more progressive professors to let me do electives in nutrition during my
fourth year.

But an interesting thing happened as we moved through our first idealistic
weeks into our final year—a time when students choose their medical residencies
and the future direction of their careers: those who were curious about nutrition
and complementary medicine dwindled from nearly eighty to less than a half-
dozen diehards. Of course, it didn't help that the standard curriculum offered no
formal CAM courses and only three one-hour lectures on nutrition.

After our clinical clerkships, the study group was forced to disband entirely.
The constant press of exams, followed by 100-hour-plus workweeks on the hospital wards drilled any remaining inquisitiveness out of us. There was little energy
left for curiosity about herbs, vitamins, meditation, acupuncture, or diet modification. My own diet suffered as I substituted tuna sandwiches from the hospital
snack bar for homemade brown rice and aduki beans.

From a class of two hundred twenty-five students, just four of us ultimately
embraced medical careers that fused complementary or nutritional approaches
with mainstream medicine. It's a small number, but still unusually high for a major
medical school. For the rest of my classmates, the scramble to pursue residencies,
set up lucrative practices, and start families left precious little time to develop even
a passing familiarity with integrative medicine.

Making Way for "Soft" Sciences

Are things different now? Yes and no. More than one hundred twenty-five medical schools now offer courses on alternative medicine. I'm proud to say that I
teach medical students at Albert Einstein about integrative medicine, though the
course is an elective and only attracts a handful of idealistic students each year. My
own medical school dean, Dr. Albert Kuperman, the very same administrator who
approved our nutrition study group twenty-five years ago, even had this to say
about integrative medicine in an article he wrote for the school newsletter *Einstein* in 2004:

> An essential feature of the integrative medicine approach is that patients are
> viewed as whole persons with minds, spiritual needs, and abundant mecha-
> nisms for innate healing. . . . Viewed from this perspective, integrative med-
> ical practice is not just about herbs, biofeedback, acupuncture, nutritional
> supplementation, imagery and visualization, ethnic and cultural healing rit-
> uals and the like. It is much more. It is about restoring trust, caring, commu-
> nication, patient participation and commitment to the relationship between
> physician and patient. And this is why we should start educating students in
> the principles, concepts, and practices of integrative medicine.[4]

But, alas, such increasing openness still hasn't translated into significant
change. For one thing, finding adequate room for "soft" sciences, like CAM and
nutrition, in crammed medical-school curricula is a little like trying to accommo-
date out-of-town Super Bowl fans—demand often overwhelms capacity. Medical
professors in pathology, genetics, anatomy, and pathophysiology literally jockey for
lecture time to present their "essential" subjects to students. Teaching "ancillary"
courses is typically seen as compromising medical-board exam scores—vital
benchmarks used for ranking medical schools. What's more, grants that schools
receive from drug companies and philanthropic groups are also more likely to
be tied to courses that reinforce mainstream medicine's emphasis on high-tech
treatments and blockbuster drugs. After all, there's little glitz—or money—in
prevention.

Even in medical schools that now clear space for "soft" subjects, graduates still
feel inadequately trained. A recent article in the *American Journal of Clinical Nutrition* notes that in 1997 (the most recent statistics available) more than 20 percent
of U.S. medical schools offered required courses in nutrition, and more than 40
percent offered elective courses in the subject.[5] Even so, 54 percent of medical
school graduates in 2002 still found their nutrition education lacking.

DEFENSIVE MEDICINE

We've all seen the headlines. America is facing a malpractice meltdown. What began as a reasonable system to guard patients against ruthless or incompetent doctors has gone awry. Physicians in many states are now retiring in droves. Emergency rooms and urgent-care centers are shutting down, and obstetrician/gynecologists are abandoning the risky business of birthing babies. In fact, doctors are joining picket lines to urge legislators to cap malpractice damage awards, and many physicians I know are having trouble paying for exorbitant insurance premiums. In one high-profile case, the husband of one of the doctors I trained with—a talented and highly ethical young dermatologist—even committed suicide after being hit with a spate of malpractice claims for unknowingly administering defective collagen injections.

Doctors are running scared, and medical innovation has suffered, particularly the practice of complementary and alternative medicine. In the past, doctors often tried a little of this and a little of that, creatively combining their limited arsenal of remedies in hopes that something would work and patients would heal. Indeed, old-time doctors were an autonomous bunch who viewed healing not only as a science but also as a personal art form. When treatments worked, medical knowledge often leapt forward. And even when treatments failed, patients were still grateful. Expectations were lower.

Of course, this "Wild West" atmosphere also yielded its share of medical excesses, including wacky experimental surgery like hysterectomy to cure female "hysteria," radiation treatment for acne, mercury therapy for syphilis, and bloodletting for release of toxic "humors." Doctors simply weren't as accountable to medical standards or authorities. The ensuing backlash eventually ushered in potent Food and Drug Administration (FDA) regulations, vigilant supervision of doctors by state medical boards, and the ever-present specter of malpractice suits.

With so many watchful eyes on them now, few mainstream M.D.s—even those who believe in the health benefits of nutrition and alternative modalities—want to risk a malpractice suit by venturing into the innovative, but largely unexplored, world of CAM. Nor can they comfortably condone a patient's decision to deviate from medicine's usual and customary practices.

Double Standard

Why do so many valid complementary and alternative therapies continue to fall outside the realm of "usual and customary?" According to an article in a recent issue of *Annals of Internal Medicine,* malpractice law typically ranks therapies into the following four categories:[6]

1. Therapies of proven safety and effectiveness.

2. Therapies of proven safety, but with inconclusive evidence of their effectiveness.

3. Therapies of proven effectiveness, but lacking confirmation of safety.

4. Therapies where evidence of both safety and efficacy is inconclusive.

Obviously, the goal of any therapy is to make it to Category 1 ("likely to work and probably won't hurt you"). These are the therapies that medical authorities look to when devising treatment guidelines that doctors follow. They're also the therapies least likely to be fingered in malpractice lawsuits.

Unfortunately, this legal rule of thumb also throws many complementary therapies squarely into the "vulnerable" pile (that is, below Category 1). Most alternative therapies simply don't rank as "sure things" because they're more difficult to control for and verify than more targeted mainstream treatments that lend themselves better to classic double-blind, placebo-controlled trials. (See Chapter 3 for more on evaluating the validity of medical studies.) Exceptions include such low-risk, well-accepted modalities as chiropractic care for low back pain, acupuncture for chemo-induced nausea and dental pain, and mind-body techniques for chronic pain and nausea, which come under Category 1.

Unfortunately, these are the exceptions. Many other well-regarded and potent CAM therapies just don't make the grade—at least not yet. These include notable Category 2 treatments ("safe but not a sure thing"), like homeopathy for seasonal allergies, massage therapy for low back pain, diet modification for cancer prevention, and acupuncture for chronic pain. Category 3 approaches ("effective but lacking conclusive safety data"), include herbal interventions like St. John's wort for depression, saw palmetto for prostatic enlargement, ginkgo biloba for dementia, and acupuncture to avert breech birth. (Obviously only the most zealous CAM devotees would dispense the kinds of risky Category 4 therapies that offer no clear-cut benefit and make malpractice litigators lick their chops.)

What many patients don't realize, though, is that several popular—and well-accepted—conventional treatments also fall below Category 1. Consider chemotherapy's sizable dangers, including its high failure rate; the frequent side effects of cholesterol-lowering statin drugs like muscle aches, liver abnormalities, and memory impairment; and even aspirin's potential to cause serious gastrointestinal bleeding. These therapies may not be perfect, but until better mainstream options come along, they often make the "A-list" of accepted treatments and find their way into care guidelines. In turn, malpractice lawyers usually steer clear of doctors who have followed the "rules."

What this double standard means is that few doctors ever learn about or try alternative treatments that might be as effective, if not more so, than mainstream therapies—and with fewer side effects. Consider the traditional Chinese herb ephedra, also known as ma huang, a tea that has been used for centuries to successfully treat asthma and allergies. Not only would it be suspect if prescribed for moderate-to-severe asthma because it falls outside the bounds of "accepted" care, but it has also now been banned by the FDA (despite the fact that a chemical copycat of ephedra, called pseudoephedrine, is still used in many best-selling, over-the-counter allergy medications like Claritin-D!). However, prednisone, mainstream medicine's asthma treatment-of-choice would pass legal muster, even though it can cause diabetes, infections, asthma, osteoporosis, cataracts, depression, and even psychosis.

With so many liability risks and mixed messages, it's amazing that physicians *ever* agree to cooperate with patients who want to try alternative approaches. My fear is that growing malpractice worries could squeeze off such cooperation entirely in the future and dampen further research into possibly important therapies.

CHECK YOUR POLICY

More than ever before, your medical insurer is making decisions about the kind of care you receive. Reining in costs is a key goal of the insurance industry, and prime targets are therapies considered experimental. Granted, cost-control is a reasonable objective as our national health expenditures soar past a trillion dollars annually. But the way healthcare insurance currently works—with doctors being paid more for providing "usual and customary" mainstream treatments—there is little incentive to try low-cost, low-tech prevention strategies, like diet modification, stress-reduction, and exercise. Instead they "scope for dollars," offering patients only insurer-sanctioned tests and procedures rather than dispensing lifestyle advice that pays little or nothing.

Yet another example of how conventional medicine rewards conformity and stifles innovation. Even doctors with an alternative bent are continually pulled into line by peer pressure, lack of CAM-training opportunities, mainstream medicine's lock-grip on defining "appropriate" care, and the fear of being sued.

Waning Idealism

Sadly, the profile of disillusionment described in "A Day in the Life" (see next page) isn't unusual. Most doctors entered medical school with a sense of purpose and idealism, ready to heal the sick and save lives, Marcus Welby–style. But once in the real world, many have found instead a medical maze of governmental regulation, piles of paperwork, health-insurer scrutiny, pressure from patients and pharmaceutical companies to prescribe the most heavily marketed brand-name drugs, and the ever-present fear of malpractice.

A Day in the Life

Long hours. Shrinking incomes. Mounds of paperwork. Demanding HMOs and rising drug company influence. Patients often grumble that doctors are short on time and bedside manner these days, but few realize the pressures most physicians face. Is it any wonder that many aren't eager to take on additional challenges by embracing CAM therapies or seeking deeper, more collaborative relationships with patients? You may not agree with their continued resistance, but that's the reality for many M.D.s. Consider this "typical" day in the life of one doctor.

6:45 A.M.

Dr. Klein rises from the breakfast table and dumps his reheated coffee down the drain. It's still dark, and his wife and the kids are asleep. No time for a real breakfast, he thinks, glancing down at his expanding waistline. "Must try to improve my diet one of these days."

Dr. Klein backs his three-year-old Honda down the driveway and heads for the hospital. Time was when he could afford a Mercedes or BMW, but not these days. Insurance companies and Medicare are squeezing reimbursements and malpractice premiums are soaring. Surgeons—like that new cardiovascular superstar Dr. Prasad with his Porsche Cayenne—might be able to charge big bucks for an operation, but in Dr. Klein's field of gastroenterology only a few procedures are reimbursable, like endoscopy and colonoscopy.

Truth is, he's working harder than ever and making less money. Even the cost of running a medical practice has skyrocketed. Once, a grandmotherly nurse/receptionist did all his paperwork and scheduling. But now with computer billing, voicemail, and complex electronic charts, he needs several full- and part-time staffers.

7:05 A.M.

Dr. Klein turns on the car radio. "Have you been a victim of Premarin, Rezulin, Propulsid, Baychol, or Vioxx?" the announcer demands. "These and other dangerous drugs have resulted in thousands of injuries and deaths. Call the law firm of Fitzsimmons and Feinstein today . . ."

It's too early to feel this way, he thinks, fighting down a pang of anxiety. Every day seems to bring more such "fear moments"—an angry message from some patient's complaining relative; a call from the insurance company announcing an audit; even a dreaded subpoena.

"Cool down," Dr. Klein mumbles, trying to quell his rising uneasiness. "It's the drug companies they're gunning for. Besides, I've got malpractice insurance—at least as long as I can afford the premiums."

7:35 A.M.

Dr. Klein hurries into the hospital to begin his teaching rounds with residents and medical students. Even though it means arriving by 7:30 two mornings a week, he actually *likes* this part of his job. Doing rounds ensures that his own patients get hospital beds—the key to his income. But it also gives him the chance to interact with young people and rekindle the intellectual excitement that drew him to medicine in the first place.

After discussing the night's admissions, Dr. Klein calls for questions. One student, an idealistic young woman, suggests that the coronary-bypass patient in Room 202 might benefit from a high-fiber Mediterranean diet instead of the macaroni and cheese/mashed potatoes and gravy/flavored gelatin that the hospital offers.

Dr. Klein checks his impatience. "Of course, in the ideal world, we'd offer patients gourmet meals," he snaps. "But with hospital costs soaring, we're lucky to get them more than a can of Ensure."

A few residents chuckle, but the young woman seems hurt.

"Look," Dr. Klein says, softening his tone. "What you say is valid, but in the *real* world of medicine, you'll discover that a majority of patients couldn't give two hoots about your nutritional and lifestyle advice; they just want to eat McDonald's and Krispy Kremes, then come in and say, 'Fix me doc.'"

10:00 A.M.

As rounds wrap up, Dr. Klein heads off to check on a few of his own patients before leaving for his office. He scans their charts, reviewing medication changes and reading consultation notes from other doctors. He's in a hurry, but these notes are important. More important than ever. Hospital watchdogs will scour them to justify sending patients home, and insurance bureaucrats will scan them to root out overcharges and unnecessary services. Moreover, every word will be scrutinized for how it might sound in court if a patient ever sues.

11:10 A.M.

Dr. Klein starts for the parking lot when a nurse runs after him. "Did you hear about your patient, Mr. Schiavoni?"

He swallows another twinge of anxiety.

"His family is ticked," she says, lowering her voice. "He was scheduled for his first radiation treatment yesterday, but I guess Southside Radiology got their signals crossed because the ambulette left him on a gurney out front . . . and the place was *closed*. Boy, is his son mad!"

11:30 A.M.

Already thirty minutes late, Dr. Klein slips through the crowded waiting room of his office and dodges a sample-toting drug representative, plying his company's latest arthritis and cholesterol-fighting drugs. No time to call Mr. Schiavoni's son now. Thankfully the day's schedule is light—only six patients before lunch and a brisk but manageable twenty-two in the afternoon. If he handles them deftly and there are no emergencies, he might finish by 5:00, put in another hour and a half for phone calls, chart dictations, and paperwork, and be home by dinnertime.

His first patient, though, upsets his plans right away by refusing the free samples of acid-blocking medication he offers for her heartburn. Instead she wants advice on foods to avoid and herbal medicines to alleviate the problem. She also seems to want some sort of emotional comfort.

Doesn't she know that he has too many patients to spend an extra fifteen minutes detailing the ideal "GERD" (gastroesophageal reflux disease) diet or offering assurances? Besides, what does he really know about herbal remedies or nurturing patients? He was trained in good old "bread-and-butter" conventional medicine with its pills, clinical studies, and "just-the-facts" precision. What do these new upscale consumers want, anyway?

12:40 P.M.

Dr. Klein considers calling out for a salad lunch, but his receptionist suggests he check out the lunchroom first. His healthy resolve melts as he gazes upon the six-foot hero sandwich, potato and macaroni salads, chips, and Cokes, courtesy of another drug company. Next to the food—competing versions of the arthritis, cholesterol-cutting and erectile dysfunction drugs he received earlier. It's getting harder and harder to keep them all straight.

1:25 P.M.

Dr. Klein's heart sinks when Mrs. Jameson greets him from the exam room table. Like so many patients these days, she's armed with paper—lists, website printouts, newspaper and magazine articles, even a mailbox solicitation for nutritional supplements—all requiring his expert opinion.

Back in medical school, his professors sometimes sarcastically referred to these obsessive patients as "hypochondriacs." But with the rise of "patient empowerment" and malpractice threats, it's now "un-PC" to wave off their complaints, even when it puts him behind schedule.

How do these patients find the time and enthusiasm to gather all this information, anyway? It isn't fair. He can't remember the last time he had a chance to surf the Web for nutrition information or sit down with a *Time* magazine article on alternative medicine. What's really scary, though, these patients sometimes actually inform *him* about new medical breakthroughs.

"Let me look at these, Mrs. Jameson," Dr. Klein says wearily, reaching for the papers. "I'll get back to you when I can."

5:15 P.M.

Twenty-one patients later, he finally gets the chance to call Mr. Schiavoni's son. Fortunately, there's no malpractice risk for him; it's the hospital's mistake. But he braces himself anyway, listening patiently as the son rants about his father's trauma in the parking lot. Dr. Klein grows increasingly annoyed (after all, mistakes happen), but he apologizes profusely and assures the son that he'll take up the matter with hospital administration.

"By the way," the son snaps, still aggravated. "I'll be transferring Dad to a better hospital. Oh, and expect to see a letter to the editor of the *Chronicle* about this mess."

6:05 P.M.

Partway through his pile of paperwork, Dr. Klein leans back in his chair and rubs his neck. Maybe he'll pack it in early today and surprise his family. The weather forecast calls for rain on Saturday anyway; he'll just stop by the office then to finish up.

Even patients seem increasingly difficult. They want more emotionally satisfying give-and-take with their physicians, more control over their healthcare decisions, and more medical options, including alternative choices—all at a time when managed-care plans expect doctors to boost efficiency and see more patients in a day.

Schooled in high-tech, disease-oriented medicine, but expected to advise patients on newer low-tech approaches that reach well beyond their training, most doctors are just plain confused and burnt out. In the next chapter we'll look at how this clash of medical cultures is wreaking havoc not just on doctors but also on their ability to communicate effectively with patients and provide top-notch care.

Medicine and Health Care in Flux

I ain't got a fever got a permanent disease
It'll take more than a doctor to prescribe a remedy
—*BAD MEDICINE* BY BON JOVI

While channel-surfing one weekend, I happened upon a curious infomercial. An attractive, sixtyish woman earnestly recounted her remarkable life story— she'd been trained as an orthopedist, but had grown disillusioned with conventional medicine, particularly after being diagnosed with invasive breast cancer.

As her website notes, "Dr. Lorraine Day was well aware that physicians are more afraid of cancer than patients are, because doctors *know* that chemotherapy, radiation, and surgery are *not* the answer to cancer."[1] By refusing these "mutilating" treatments and turning instead to natural means, Dr. Day claims not only to have cured her "terminal" cancer, but also now believes alternative therapies ("God's natural remedies") are the key to healing anyone with cancer.

I was impressed by Dr. Day's confidence and self-assuredness. When counseling *my* patients with cancer, I wish I could bring even a fraction of her belief in the infallible power of diet, supplements, and prayer to my wellness advice. But experience treating cancer and other challenging medical maladies has taught me that it's not usually so easy to eschew conventional treatments with full confidence that alternatives are the *only* answer.

Of course, on the other side, self-proclaimed "quackbusters" also paint with overly broad brushstrokes. They holler about CAM's "unscientific" claims, and point to an epidemic of scientific illiteracy in America. If only the public were better educated, they lament. Then belief in "natural" cures would simply melt away under the withering beam of intelligent scrutiny.

What troubles me most about pronouncements from each of these warring "camps" is that good health care shouldn't proceed from an ideology. What we need is pragmatism. Questioning complementary and alternative medicine under

17

the guise of "rationalism" is no less biased than warning patients against the "slash, burn, poison" of conventional treatments.

In this chapter we'll take a look at this current clash of medical cultures. We'll explore their attempts to merge, as well as the problem areas where integration remains stuck. We'll also explore the fallout from this process, including rising communication barriers between doctors and patients who increasingly speak separate languages.

MAINSTREAM MEDICINE IN CRISIS

No doubt about it. Complementary medicine—the integration of conventional and alternative therapies—is moving beyond the fringes to become a recognized movement. This growing receptivity is being partly fueled by the baby-boom generation. We're the first generation to be born into relative prosperity, fed on the certainty that scientific advancements would extend our life spans and ease every discomfort. In fact, we may be the first generation to say no to the ravages of aging. Indeed, our expectations about what's possible have catapulted many of us into the ranks of the "worried well"—those of us who are basically healthy but either have a family history of disease or unexplained symptoms that don't respond to treatment. Fifty-five is the new thirty-five, as the saying goes. And unlike our parents and grandparents before us, we've sought to stave off wrinkles and disease by popping vitamins and Viagra—anything that might enhance our health and longevity—with the same experimental fervor that we once sampled hash brownies and blotter acid in the 1960s and 1970s.

Unfortunately, the promise of "better living through chemistry" (particularly all those high-tech drugs and treatments we grew up embracing) hasn't fully materialized. Study after study shows that modern medicine is a veritable "Jurassic Park" of unforeseen consequences and treatments run amok. Witness the recent flap over female hormone replacement therapy and widely publicized concerns about overuse of antidepressants in children. One result has been a higher populist demand than ever for gentler, more effective alternatives.

Add to this the fact that we're spending more money, per capita, on health care than any other country in the world. Yet our health statistics and mortality rates lag far behind many other developed countries.

Consider these disturbing numbers from a recent study, which concluded that doctors cause 225,000 hospital deaths each year due to errors and adverse drug reactions—the third leading cause of death in the United States after heart disease and cancer![2]

- 7,000 medication errors in hospitals
- 12,000 unnecessary surgeries

- 20,000 "other" errors in hospitals
- 80,000 infections in hospitals
- 106,000 non-error negative effects of drugs

Such statistics might be acceptable if Americans realized better health, the study notes. But that's not the case. In a recent comparison of thirteen industrialized nations, the United States ranked twelfth (second from the bottom) on sixteen health indicators, including infant mortality and low birth-weight (we rank last on both).

Consider also that our ability to finance health care in the next few decades is increasingly uncertain. In fact, treating common diseases, like heart disease and Alzheimer's disease, which will soon afflict baby boomers big time, threatens to bankrupt our healthcare system.

It's no wonder then that even experts are warming to the idea of using low-tech, low-cost CAM therapies in conjunction with high-tech conventional treatments, not only to improve overall health but to also cut the nation's future medical bills. As another study recently suggested, something as simple as taking a daily multivitamin to protect against diseases of aging could save Medicare $1.6 billion over five years.[3] The following are some advantages of using a CAM approach:

- "Holistic," patient-centered care
- Lower toxicity and fewer side effects
- Emphasis on doctor-patient relationship
- Engenders hope
- Focus on prevention
- Addresses concerns ignored by mainstream medicine
- Patient is an active participant in care

Blurring the Battle Lines

A few progressive doctors are also pushing for more use of complementary and alternative therapies as they seek better ways to prevent and treat disease, as well as satisfy the desires of their increasingly savvy patients for more communication and better partnerships. When faced with a choice of residencies after medical school twenty-five years ago, I was tempted to apply for a Preventive Medicine residency. But I learned to my disappointment that "preventive medicine" consisted of little more than making sure that basic sanitation needs were being met in impoverished communities and ensuring kids were getting vaccinated.

Certainly, great strides have been made in the field of preventive medicine in the last quarter century. In cardiology we're now using cholesterol tests and statin drugs to ward off heart problems. Bone-density screening and bone-strengthening medications are now widely deployed to forestall osteoporosis. But what I was looking for then, and what many CAM doctors like me incorporate into their practices now, is a more definitive approach using our best knowledge about diet, exercise, and supplemental nutrients. We constantly strive to meet the needs of our patients who are eager to optimize their health and deploy pre-emptive strategies against cancer, brain degeneration, or just the energy decline that comes with stress and aging.

I recently received this e-mail from one of my radio listeners:

Dear Dr. Hoffman:

I just had my annual physical. My fasting blood sugar was 114 . . . and hemoglobin A1c was 7. . . . I was told I'm borderline diabetic and should go on a special diet . . . but was not told what kind of diet to follow. Please advise . . . need feedback on diet specifics.

Mrs. H. G.

I think this e-mail underscores one of the key limitations of conventional medicine, which misses such critical "prevention" opportunities by not specifying what type of diet might halt the onset of non-insulin dependent diabetes. How unfortunate that a person sees her physician, gets a warning, but receives no emotional support or specific tools to avert an impending health crisis, and has to resort to writing a radio doctor for crucial health information.

If this patient were in a complementary medicine practice like mine (Chapter 3 explores this in greater depth), she'd receive not only detailed diet information, but also suggestions for supplements, exercise, and a comprehensive evaluation of her cardiovascular risk. That might include tests rarely done in conventional medical settings, like an EBT (electron beam tomography) scan of her coronary arteries and a high-sensitivity C-reactive protein test (see Chapter 6 for more on cardiovascular prevention). Then we'd discuss her options and work with her to devise a diabetes prevention plan tailored to her specific health needs and personal goals.

Keeping the Baby with the Bath Water

Of course, none of this is meant to denigrate mainstream health care. The forte of conventional medicine has always been crisis intervention (see the inset "Which Approach to Take—Conventional, Alternative, or Both?" on page 22). When I fractured my shoulder ten years ago, I asked to be brought to a high-tech emergency room for definitive orthopedic care. Similarly, mainstream medicine is the go-to place for cardiac emergencies, acute abdominal crises (appendicitis, diverticulitis, gall bladder), critical cancer interventions, and stroke. Even in HIV infection, modern medicine has made undeniable progress.

But as the chart indicates, conventional health care is only partially effective against many major medical problems, like cancer and hypertension, and has little to offer for marginalized, chronic concerns, such as fatigue, frequent minor respiratory infections like sinus problems and frequent colds, chronic back pain, headaches, irritable bowel syndrome, and osteoarthritis. Even where conventional therapies do offer some answers (as in the case of asthma, cancer, colitis, Crohn's disease, eczema, depression, and anxiety) their impact often falls far short of the ideal level of wellness that most patients seek. In fact, many patients end up preferring the condition itself to the high cost and unwanted side effects often linked with mainstream treatments.

In my experience, integrating alternative measures with conventional approaches ups the chance of success by capitalizing on the strengths of both. And patients who use natural therapies often develop better skills for managing their own conditions, yielding a sense of empowerment.

Two Approaches May Be Better Than One

Fortunately, mainstream medicine is also waking up to the idea that two healing approaches may be better than one. Many therapies once considered unconventional—or even downright quackery—are well on their way to becoming mainstream (see "From 'Holistic' to Conventional" on page 23).

Even insurers are embracing the complementary model. A recent *Wall Street Journal* article noted that 47 percent of employees with health benefits had acupuncture coverage in 2004, up from 33 percent in 2002.[4] Chiropractic coverage increased to 87 percent from 79 percent.

Indeed, acceptance of alternative self-healing and prevention strategies is now so widespread that nutritional supplements and herbs are nearly "staples" of the American diet. A recent survey found that 52 percent of adults now augment their diets with supplements, compared to only 23 percent in 1970.[5]

As a result of all this interest, more mainstream doctors are also softening to the idea of complementary and alternative medicine. My aunt recently began seeing a new doctor. While discussing nutrition and alternative medicine with him, she happened to announce that her nephew was a radio doctor.

"Oh, that guy," the doctor said. "I used to *hate* him! My patients would come in all the time asking me about something that Dr. Hoffman said on the radio. Used to drive me crazy!"

WHICH APPROACH TO TAKE—CONVENTIONAL, ALTERNATIVE, OR BOTH?			
Condition	Conventional	Both	Alternative
Alzheimer's Disease		X	
Anxiety/Depression		X	
Cancer Prevention			X
Cancer Treatment		X	
Chronic Back Pain			X
Chronic Fatigue			X
Diabetes		X	
Fibromyalgia			X
GERD		X	
Headaches		X	
Heart Attack	X		
Heart Disease Prevention		X	
HIV/AIDS		X	
Hypertension		X	
Irritable Bowel			X
Mild Infections			X
Obesity			X
Osteoarthritis		X	
Osteoporosis		X	
Seasonal Allergies		X	
Syndrome X			X
Trauma	X		
Ulcers		X	

"But why do you say you 'used to' hate him?" my aunt asked, puzzled.

"Well, I finally listened a couple of times, and he did make a fair amount of sense."

Not exactly a ringing endorsement, but better than the resistance and outright disdain that have come my way in the past. In fact, some conventional doctors are now moving beyond mere tolerance and are beginning to offer CAM therapies themselves or at least are allowing patients to try complementary and alternative medicine or referring them to CAM providers.

One reason is to help steer patients clear of harmful treatments and adverse interactions with conventional treatments. Yet many doctors still wish they knew more—a major reason why I wrote this book.

According to a recent study, nearly one-quarter of 276 Colorado physicians said they'd used CAM, and roughly two-thirds said they had patients who used CAM.[6] Yet only one-third of the doctors said they felt "somewhat comfortable" discussing use of these therapies with their patients, and only 35 percent said they had "somewhat positive" feelings about such discussions. The remaining physicians either felt "uncomfortable or neutral" or had "negative or neutral" feelings.

The study's authors concluded that such discomfort points to a CAM knowledge gap rather than outright opposition to alternative therapies, since 84 percent of the doctors indicated they were interested in learning more.

They urged more CAM education in medical schools, residency programs, and continuing education courses for practicing doctors. Plus, they recommended that patients do their part to ensure proper dialogue and minimize adverse treatment interactions by telling their physicians what complementary and alternative modalities they're using, as well as seeking out CAM and conventional practitioners who are willing to partner with each other.

Miscommunication and Missed Opportunities

Obviously, the American healthcare system is in the process of transformation, situated somewhere between the old-style conventional model and the newer integrative model. The good news is that growing acceptance of CAM therapies has

FROM "HOLISTIC" TO CONVENTIONAL	
Treatment	Condition
Acupuncture	Headache, Nausea of Pregnancy
Biofeedback	Anxiety, Headache, Irritable Bowel Syndrome, Pelvic Floor Dysfunction
Coenzyme Q_{10}	Parkinson's Disease
DHEA	Lupus
Fish Oil	Heart Disease, Depression, Bipolar Disorder, Arthritis
Glucosamine	Arthritis
Hypnosis	Dental Anesthesia, Irritable Bowel Syndrome
Meditation	Hypertension
Natural Hormones	Menopause
Probiotics	Diarrhea, Irritable Bowel Syndrome

handed more doctors an expanded arsenal of treatments and has resulted in better medical care for more patients. But the shift has also brought its share of confusion. Medicine is in a state of flux, and nothing has taken a harder hit than the sacred bond between doctors and patients.

Conventional doctors may be curious about CAM treatments, as the previous study suggests, but many still don't know where to find more information or they lack time to sift through the CAM literature (which admittedly is often contradictory and in flux itself).

Indeed, most struggle just to keep pace with new findings in *conventional* medicine, often sticking with the tried-and-true procedures they learned in medical school or the strategies suggested by colleagues. The fact is, many not only fail to try complementary and alternative therapies, but they also fail to adopt newly recommended mainstream treatments. One study by the Rand Corporation, a Santa Monica, California, think-tank, reported recently that, on average, American adults only receive about half of the care recommended by conventional treatment guidelines.[7] For example, about 76 percent of diabetics aren't getting routine glycosylated hemoglobin A1c screening (essential to halt complications, like kidney failure) and only 45 percent of heart-attack patients are on beta blockers, which cut the risk of premature death.

Even when doctors do follow established guidelines, patients don't always receive good care. As we've seen, bias runs rampant in mainstream medicine. Doctors and patients are constantly bombarded by exhortations in medical journals, magazine ads, and commercials to try various drugs. Even studies published in venerable medical journals are often biased. Head-to-head comparisons of one manufacturer's drugs are cleverly crafted to trump competing drugs, and conflicts of interest abound. Many "independent" researchers are actually on the payroll of pharmaceutical companies.

Even "gold standard" drugs often turn out to be less golden than their published studies and marketing hype suggest—sometimes with fatal consequences. Witness the pain drug Vioxx. One day it's in medicine cabinets everywhere and the next whisked off the market because of deadly side effects. Merck & Co. executives were excoriated for ignoring early evidence of potential heart problems among Vioxx users; rather than commissioning a few relatively inexpensive studies to validate its safety, they barraged the media with hundreds of millions of dollars of direct-to-consumer ads promoting it.

Even profitable Viagra got a speeding ticket recently when the FDA demanded Pfizer withdraw its popular "Wild Thing—He's Back!" ad (the one where the guy grows Viagra-purple horns). Regulators correctly noted that the clinical trials leading to Viagra's FDA approval as an erectile dysfunction treatment didn't also guarantee it would restore guys to their former youthful "studliness." Though the claim wasn't necessarily deadly, studies show that when erectile dysfunction drugs prove disappointing, feelings of inadequacy and depression can be compounded.

Such tumult in the medical marketplace has propelled more patients to take control of their own care, leaving many conventional physicians unsure about their role as dispensers of medical knowledge. More waiting rooms are now filled with highly informed medical consumers seeking to partner with their doctors. They want to explore all promising treatments, both mainstream and alternative, and connect emotionally.

To physicians, these patients seem needy and demanding. They expect a lot of attention, but are all too quick to question authority and battle doctors for control of medicine. To patients, though, such physicians come off as distant and stodgy, even arrogant. Many walk away entirely from mainstream medicine seeking better partnerships or they neglect to mention the alternative treatments

HOW OPEN IS YOUR DOCTOR TO INTEGRATIVE MEDICINE?

EXCELLENT

Doctor's Responses: "I encourage you to participate in your care by researching and applying alternative approaches to your condition—let's talk about what might be most helpful and compatible with your conventional treatment. If you prefer, we'll use standard medicine only as a last resort."

Grade: Excellent

Suggested Action: Congratulations! You've found an ideal "health coach" who will supervise and support your wellness efforts.

GOOD

Doctor's Responses: "I'm somewhat familiar with these approaches. I believe some work, some don't, and some could be downright harmful. I'll try to get information on how the alternatives you're taking could interact with my standard treatments—my goal is just to keep you safe."

Grade: Good

Suggested Action: Encourage your doctor to partner with you and provide detailed info on CAM treatments to bridge her/his knowledge gap.

FAIR

Doctor's Responses: "I'm frankly skeptical about these 'alternatives' you're using, and admit I don't know much about them. I guess you can try them, but keep me informed, and I'll alert you to any possible interactions."

Grade: Marginal

Suggested Action: Inform your doctor that you would welcome a more accepting attitude. The situation is salvageable—but you will have to be tactful and proactive.

POOR

Doctor's Responses: "There you go about those *alternatives* again! When are you going to just accept that they're dangerous, unproven, and mostly rip-offs! If you keep on trying to play doctor, I'm afraid I won't be able to keep on treating you."

Grade: Unsatisfactory

Suggested Action: Vote with your feet!

they're using for fear of disapproval. Less assertive patients simply clam up—put off by doctors' increasingly brusque bedside manner and shorthand use of "medicalese." Not only are they afraid to speak up and ask for simpler, less technical explanations, but also they willingly abdicate all responsibility for their own care.

The unfortunate result in each case is the same: patients fail to receive the best care available to them and doctor-patient relationships fall far short of the caring and mutually satisfying exchanges they could be. (Chapter 3 explores how a fully developed CAM approach might improve medical care and strengthen physician-patient bonds.) To get a sense of how open your own doctor is to using non-traditional therapies, see "How Open Is Your Doctor to Integrative Medicine?" on page 25.

A CHALLENGE FOR HOLISTIC DOCTORS

Conventional doctors aren't the only ones facing obstacles to good patient relations. As medicine changes, holistic physicians are encountering their share of communication mishaps, too. Granted, they're different from those in conventional settings, but they are equally likely to result in less-than-optimal medical care and unsatisfying patient-physician encounters.

I spotted this breathy alumni greeting from a member of my own graduating class in a recent edition of my college magazine. I think it epitomizes some of the high-striving, peripatetic Boomer-types I grew up with and now often see as patients—sometimes with mixed results.

Class of '74

D.B. . . . Graduated from Yale Med School in '77 and Harvard Law in '89. He is a professional polo player (!), plays jazz piano, and represents Steinway and Bosendorfer pianos. He's a practicing Tibetan Buddhist, collects Asian Art, and has lived in recent years in Big Sur, Calif., Tucson, and Jamaica. He lives in Easton, Connecticut, and is proud of having attended the college.

Expectations loom large for these perfectionist strivers. I recently met with a young "worried-well" patient who came expressly to New York from her home in Bermuda to see me. During a recent trip to Italy, she'd experienced an "allergic reaction" after eating several seafood meals. This included a bizarre and scary set of symptoms that got worse with each exposure, including heart-pounding, a sensation of breathlessness, dizziness, and tingling and numbness of her lips and fingers and toes. At first she saw an Italian doctor, who gave her an antihistamine, but the symptoms recurred, and she was rushed to an emergency room for extensive tests.

I asked if she'd ever had a throat-closing sensation or if her tongue or face had ever swelled (characteristics of a potentially life-threatening anaphylactic reaction). She hadn't. I also asked about other food allergies and her family's history of allergy—all standard questions. Again, no to both.

Even more disconcerting, her symptoms (including frequent headaches, dizziness, a "sick feeling" in her stomach, PMS bloating, and a "burning sensation" on her skin) had persisted despite eliminating all seafood from her diet. Now the symptoms were occurring without rhyme or reason, seemingly provoked by many foods. She'd seen several doctors in Bermuda, and when they failed to uncover any conclusive causes, consulted more specialists in Miami and New York. She was tested for Lyme disease, multiple sclerosis, colitis, cardiac arrhythmias, autoimmune conditions like lupus, even ovarian cancer—all to no avail.

When conventional doctors failed to help, she'd turned to a series of complementary physicians. One doctor tried to "desensitize" her to fish and other foods with homeopathic drops under the tongue. These helped some, she said, but the symptoms came back. Another put her on a series of detoxification fasts, which also helped for a while, but she felt weak and had to abandon the "detox" when her periods stopped. The next doctor told her she had mercury toxicity (my tests revealed she didn't) and gave her a popular mercury-chelating formula. When her symptoms got worse, he told her this was natural during a purge of toxic metals. She hung in for a while, but ultimately quit. Yet another assured her that high doses of intravenous magnesium would make her feel better. At first, they did, but then, like everything else, they stopped working. A final doctor diagnosed candida (a fungal infection) and cut her intake of sugar and fermented foods and prescribed an antifungal medication. Still no luck.

Promising Too Much

Clinical dilemmas like this come up often for "holistic" practitioners. One of the drawbacks of our medical style is that, while it's "patient-centered," it also sometimes encourages "somatization"—a recognized psychiatric malady in which patients seek treatment for several ongoing symptoms that typically impair their ability to function from day to day. Often, no medical syndrome exists to explain them. And when one does, it isn't usually critical enough to account for the severity or persistence of the complaints.

Conventional M.D.s tend to label these kinds of challenging symptoms "psychological." However, alternative practitioners often fall prey to the opposite by elevating such disparate and bewildering physical problems to the status of missed "clues." For them, symptoms indicate an underlying (and usually medically controversial) condition, like hypoglycemia, food intolerance, nutritional deficiencies, or reactions to harmful environmental agents. The downside of this approach is that it can sometimes produce unintended results, such as the following:

- Delay of appropriate diagnosis, therapy
- Interactions with conventional treatments
- Overuse of medical resources
- "Rube Goldberg" effect
- Side effects/adverse effects
- Somatization
- Susceptibility to placebo influences
- "Tell me it ain't so" medicine
- Unrealistic expectations

When this kind of detective work pays off, the results can verge on the mirac-
ulous. When it's misguided, though, the outcome reinforces somatization and fortifies the patient's denial about the disorder's true psychological underpinnings. In
many cases, a cure might be achieved with something as simple as talk therapy or
relaxation techniques (maybe coupled with a short course of medication). But
instead the patient and practitioner end up fashioning an elaborate "Rube Goldberg" contraption of arcane therapies.

My young patient had all the trappings of a psychological disorder that was
either triggered by an allergic reaction—or simply developed spontaneously. I
considered gently pointing this out, but she talked on relentlessly, insisting that I
pay close attention to every nuance of her complex syndrome.

Finally, I interjected, explaining that I needed more time to study her records,
perhaps talk to her other doctors, and order a few more tests of my own. In the
meantime, I suggested she speak to our nutritionist about a hypoglycemia diet to
avoid wide swings in blood sugar, and that she limit foods known to trigger his-
tamine production that could exacerbate her allergy symptoms. I also suggested
that she continue her magnesium drips to calm her nerves.

"You know," I ventured, hesitating. "After everything you've been through
have you considered the possibility that anxiety might now be playing a part in
your symptoms?"

The patient's expression darkened: "So, you think this is all in my head?" she
snapped. "I assure you these symptoms are very *real,* they're *physical.*"

"I don't doubt they're real," I plowed on (there's no doubt that psychosomatic
symptoms *feel* the same to sufferers as physical symptoms). "But it might help to
talk to someone about coping with your illness or getting help with relaxation."

"Well, I don't think that's relevant," she said, producing a three-month symptom diary, detailing her every bodily sensation for the past ninety days.

Needless to say, she wasn't happy when I said I couldn't extend our appointment beyond the promised hour and a half. Ultimately, she didn't pursue treatment with me, but her case illustrates the inherent pitfalls of a CAM approach that promises some patients too much.

BETWEEN TWO WORLDS

Other patients find themselves caught in the paradigm shift—pulled in two directions by competing views of healing. They may be tempted by CAM's promise and high-touch, low-tech approach, but are afraid to entirely forgo the security and sense of belonging afforded by mainstream medicine. In trying to straddle both worlds they often find themselves torn between "warring" practitioners who can't—or won't—collaborate.

One of my long-term patients, Mrs. C., recently came in after being diagnosed with an aggressive form of breast cancer. I informed her that her nutritional treatment plan would depend on the results of surgery, which I encouraged her to undertake. (Some patients who dread drastic conventional intervention invoke me as their court of last resort to "tell 'em it ain't so." But I recommend treatments based on their ability to help patients, not whether they wear the "alternative" or "conventional" label). I suggested some general nutritional support for surgical healing, and told her to avoid supplements that might interfere with anesthesia or put her at risk for perioperative bleeding. (See Chapter 11 for more on preparing for surgery and recovery.)

I also prescribed a nutritional support program to ease damage from chemo and radiation, at the same time omitting certain nutrients thought to interfere with conventional cancer therapy. Phase 2 after chemo and radiation would be a broader-based supplement program aimed at immune restoration and long-term prevention of cancer recurrence. I told her to "lighten up" on her stringent vegan diet because chemo and radiation typically dampen appetite, which could cause her already marginal weight to plummet. I wished her luck and told her to see me again in a few weeks.

The patient returned about six months later, looking decidedly emaciated. I asked if she'd adhered to my supplement and diet recommendations, but she sheepishly admitted she hadn't been taking the supplements. Apparently, her oncologist had referred her to a registered dietician who feared that the few supplements I'd suggested might interfere with the cancer-fighting effects of radiation and chemo. My patient was left feeling intensely conflicted.

She had confidence in me, but after all, the R.D. worked for one of the nation's largest and most prestigious cancer hospitals. The "party line" there was that cancer patients should take a single weak commercial multivitamin, ubiquitous at drugstores. She opted for the one-a-day vitamin.

Poisoning the Well

Several things bothered me about this encounter—and it really epitomizes the transition in medicine that often tugs at patients. I'm not one to pull rank, but I'm a physician trained in internal medicine with more than a passing knowledge of up-to-date approaches to cancer. Not only that, I'm steeped in decades of nutrition study, including cancer nutrition. Granted, a legitimate debate continues on how effective supplements are in preventing and treating cancer, and a sizeable, though diminishing, sector of conservative cancer nutritionists adamantly believe that certain nutrients—antioxidants especially—can take the punch out of hard-hitting cancer treatments. But it strikes me as a breach of professional etiquette to overrule a patient's doctor—essentially "poisoning the well" of potentially beneficial nutritional therapies. Why not simply pick up the phone to hear my rationale for recommending all those supplements?

I could see by my patient's frightened expression that her confidence in my nutritional recommendations was probably permanently damaged. In her mind, her best chance of escaping the ravages of cancer now lay with the cancer center. It was enough to make her toe the line and stop taking all my supplements. She simply didn't have the stuffings in her frail condition to be embroiled in a contentious tug-of-war between me and the oncology team.

"Look," I told her, backing off, "I'm not going to pressure you—you're in a tough enough position just dealing with your cancer."

She eased noticeably. "But," I added, "I *am* really concerned about your weight loss." She'd dropped nearly twenty pounds since the start of chemo and radiation.

She finally admitted that she was still following a strict vegetarian diet, mainly because she'd read somewhere that ultra-low fat, low-protein foods could curb the growth of cancer.

We discussed studies showing a link between calorie restriction and cancer prevention. But as I noted, researchers still don't know whether fat and protein are the culprits or whether excess carbs are to blame. "Besides," I added, "you have to keep up your strength during cancer treatment to overcome the debilitating effects."

She finally agreed to let me call her dietician and try to get her on board with my recommendations. The dietician sounded a little taken aback, but I immediately defused the situation by admitting there were a lot of nutritional controversies to be solved in the cancer field. I also told her I supported the patient's choice right now to take a conservative approach.

"Thanks for understanding," the dietician replied, a bit apologetically. "That's the way we do things here; we're just waiting until a few more studies come in, you know how it is."

"I understand," I reassured her. "But I'm concerned that Mrs. C. is still on a calorically inadequate diet." I described her alarming weight loss, and the dietician immediately agreed she needed more calories and variety in her diet. We also agreed to cooperate in the future and ended the call cordially.

Three months later Mrs. C. came in again. To me, she looked as skinny as ever, but there was more color in her face and resolve in her stride. I saw from her chart that she'd regained nearly twenty pounds.

"It really worked!" she exclaimed. "I put more fat in my diet, even added a little animal protein, and I feel better. That dietician even has me eat a serving of premium Haagen Dazs every night!"

With her chemo and radiation now over, I suggested she add a few more cancer-preventive and immune-supportive nutrients, which she agreed to do.

If only every attempt to blend CAM and conventional medicine ended so well. Ideally, I would've preferred to collaborate fully with her oncologist and dietician to develop a comprehensive healing plan. But unfortunately that's still quite rare. As we'll see in the next chapter, my hope is that medicine ultimately works through its growing pains, combining the best conventional therapies with the best alternative treatments for a fully integrated approach. This would not only allow doctors the freedom to try *all* promising therapies (either on their own or in conjunction with a team of CAM practitioners), but patients would receive the full complement of care they deserve, including emotionally enriching partnerships with their doctors.

Creating a New Vision of Medical Practice

The greatest discovery of any generation is that human beings can alter their lives by altering the attitudes of their minds.
—ALBERT SCHWEITZER

Dear Dr. Hoffman:

I can't come to your center, but I would like to let you know that after reading your article on "Mitral Valve Prolapse" (MVP, a type of heart murmur), I am in awe.[1] I have suffered from panic attacks (a little recognized symptom of MVP) for years. All my doctors do is dope me up . . . they treat me as if I were a hypochondriac. It's so frustrating. Now I have hope that I can do something about my health. Just knowing I am not crazy is a relief.

Jamie, West Virginia

I receive letters and e-mails like this constantly because of my books and my radio program. Time and again I hear, "I need a doctor who will listen and care—someone who will take me seriously and quit throwing pills at me."

What always amazes me is that, though I've never met these people, their lives are so touched by what I've written or said on the air. To me, this belies a tremendous unmet need among patients for comfort, compassion, and a "holistic" approach to their care—a need that's not being met by the current medical system.

A typical case from my practice illustrates how a conventional medical approach leaves some patients "high and dry," and how complementary intervention can often attend to their real inner concerns. It's a comprehensive approach, including strong doctor/patient partnering, that I hope will eventually take hold throughout the entire medical system and not just in a few CAM practices like mine.

MELDING OLD AND NEW

Jack, a classic forty-five-year-old, "worried-well" patient and active commodities trader, decided to see me about ongoing chest pressure after conventional doctors failed to find anything wrong. Jack first noticed vague discomfort during his morning runs, shortly after his older brother died suddenly of a massive heart attack while playing squash. Both his father and grandfather had also died young of heart disease.

The painful sensations became more frequent, first occurring at work and then at night, often waking him from sleep. Alarmed, Jack scheduled an appointment with his internist, who examined him and performed an ECG (electrocardiogram). The results were normal, but the internist sent Jack to a cardiologist anyway—just to be safe.

The cardiologist didn't find anything wrong either, but in the interest of caution decided to put Jack on aspirin and a heart-protective medication called a beta blocker. He also scheduled him for a stress test, advising him to abstain from exercise until the test results were in and avoid all unnecessary stress—not an easy feat in Jack's pressure-cooker job.

The medication seemed to work for a while, but then the chest sensations resurfaced. Jack began feeling preoccupied at work and missed a couple of key bids. He noticed his memory and concentration were off. Was it the effect of the medication? He called the cardiologist, but he couldn't come to the phone. However, a nurse urged him to stay on his medication. Jack decided to take a few days off.

The day of the stress test Jack began striding on the treadmill but was quickly winded—a far cry from how he'd felt just a few weeks before.

Even more alarming, his results came back abnormal, indicating a possible blockage. The cardiologist ordered a cardiac catheterization to confirm it. He explained that during the procedure a wire would be inserted into Jack's groin, then threaded up to his heart to take pictures. He also assured Jack that if any blockage was found, he'd clear it right then and possibly put in a couple of heart stents (wire mesh tubes used to prop open newly cleared arteries).

Oddly—and disconcertingly—the cardiac catheterization showed *no* blockage. The cardiologist took Jack off the beta blocker and assured him, "It's not cardiac." However, he recommended that Jack continue taking aspirin, as well as a cholesterol-lowering statin drug "for protection."

Jack was left more confused than ever by the mixed messages, particularly when his chest discomfort continued. He revisited his internist, who referred him to a gastroenterologist to test for possible stomach irritation or gastroesophageal reflux disease (GERD). Again, the tests came back normal, but the gastroenterologist still felt compelled to prescribe a powerful prescription acid blocker. The new pill *changed* Jack's chest discomfort slightly, but it remained.

Even with his supposed clean bill of health, Jack continued feeling anxious about his grim family history and the nagging feeling in his chest. Fearful of resuming exercise, he gained nearly twenty pounds. When he returned to his internist and revealed his ongoing fears, the doctor assured him there was nothing wrong with him physically and offered him a sample of Paxil for his "anxiety."

Essential Healing Work

That's when Jack decided to consult me. Like so many patients I see, he'd been thoroughly "worked up" medically, but left hanging emotionally. I spent much of that first visit just listening to him—making sure he felt heard and understood. I also tried to *reassure* him by interpreting the results of all those medical tests and *empower* him to take control of his health again by outlining some preventive measures he could enlist to cut his heart-disease risk.

We began by addressing Jack's legitimate concern about the health of his heart. Jack was having chest pains, he was still afraid to exercise, and he was taking a statin drug, perhaps unnecessarily. I took him off the statin for a while so we could properly assess his cholesterol and cardiovascular risk without it. (For a list of appropriate heart-disease tests and treatments, see Chapters 4 and 6.) I also suggested Jack take an EBT (electron beam tomography) heart scan to determine if he had any coronary artery calcification. An EBT scan often provides an early warning snapshot of small plaque accumulations that normal stress tests and catheterization tests may miss.

Next, I questioned Jack about his diet. I discovered that he often bolstered his energy by downing cups of coffee and cans of Coke, which may have sent his blood sugar levels into the stratosphere, followed by an inevitable plummet. Besides their corrosive effect on his esophagus (a possible cause of his chest discomfort), caffeinated beverages were probably also boosting his anxiety—another possible cause of phantom chest pain. When a five-hour glucose tolerance test revealed that Jack had hypoglycemia (low blood sugar), we put him on a low-refined carbohydrate regimen, and tapered his caffeine.

The good news was that Jack's EBT scan showed *zero* calcification, indicating clean coronary arteries. While his cholesterol was a little high after stopping the statin medication, a test of his "bad" LDL (low-density lipoprotein) cholesterol revealed that it was a less risky type and would likely be responsive to dietary modification and exercise. I explained to Jack that statins weren't immediately necessary, but he'd need a good diet and exercise regimen, as well as certain heart-protective supplements to overcome his strong family history of heart disease.

Jack was elated. It was as if a pall had been lifted from him. His vague chest pains disappeared with the diet change. He lost most of the weight that he'd gained and confidently resumed his exercise. In addition, he felt more energetic than he'd felt in ten years. When Jack returned several months later, his cholesterol was down a solid 80 points, and his chest pains were a thing of the past.

THE ROAD TO STRONG DOCTOR-PATIENT PARTNERSHIPS

A recent *Wall Street Journal Online*/Harris Interactive poll seems to confirm what Jack came to realize and what holistic physicians have known for years: patients don't necessarily want dazzling scientific virtuosity from their doctors. They want better communication.[2]

According to the poll, 85 percent of respondents felt that treating a patient with dignity and respect is an extremely important quality in a doctor; 84 percent cited listening carefully and being easy to talk to as important attributes; and only 58 percent said that having "a lot of experience treating patients with your medical condition" is extremely important.

Respondents also indicated that their major reason for changing doctors in the last five years was because they weren't being listened to enough (14 percent). This ranked well above having a doctor who didn't keep abreast of the latest medical breakthroughs (5 percent).

Such findings make many mainstream doctors uneasy. A few years back, I attended a conference on "anti-aging medicine" which explored innovative approaches to forestalling disease and promoting longevity. During a break, I sat down to lunch with an old friend, a veteran complementary physician like myself. Across the table sat a young physician we didn't know.

"Your first conference?" I ventured.

He nodded.

"Interesting, isn't it?" my friend said.

"Well, yes . . . actually, it's a little mind-blowing," the young doctor admitted. "I've never attended a conference like this . . . so many new ideas and approaches . . . I'm not quite sure what to make of it all."

As we talked, I learned that he was a gastroenterologist searching for new ways to deal with "problem patients" who eluded conventional diagnosis or treatment. My friend and I described our complementary practices, and his eyes widened.

"You mean you *actually* see patients who have *absolutely nothing wrong with them clinically* and then offer suggestions about what to do?" he asked in amazement.

"That's right," we said almost simultaneously. "You've heard of preventive medicine?"

"Well, sure . . ." he said, nervously picking at his food. I could see he was intrigued, but obviously not fully convinced that our approach was the way to go. The conversation lapsed after that.

"Give 'Em an Inch"

Certainly, he's not alone in his discomfort. Many conventional physicians are baffled by "worried well" patients like Jack—patients who seem to need and want more than the high-tech tests and drugs they learned to dispense in medical school. They're also more than a little afraid. As the old saying goes, "Give 'em an inch, and they'll take a mile." In other words, surrender to patients' craving for intimacy and consolation, and the only thing you're likely to encourage is hypochondriacal dependency, not better health.

Recall the famous scene in Woody Allen's film *Hannah and Her Sisters* where Woody, who is suffering from headaches, examines a CAT scan of his brain with his doctor. The doctor is actually portrayed by a real M.D. instead of a professional actor to capture the realism of the encounter. The dialogue goes something like this:

Woody: Doc, what do you see?

Doctor: Nothing. Nothing, really.

Woody: What do you mean "nothing"?

Doctor: Well, it's probably nothing, but of course there are other possibilities.

Woody: What? What?

Doctor: Well, there is this funny little irregularity over here, and it's probably nothing . . .

Woody: What do you mean?

Doctor: But of course, it could be an abnormal blood vessel, or else it could be . . .

Woody: What?

Doctor: A brain tumor, it could be a brain tumor but, of course, that's extremely unlikely.

And just like that, Woody is off to the races, tragically contemplating his own demise.

Thinking Out Loud

Why do so many doctors discuss dire medical possibilities with patients and issue cold medical verdicts as if patients were out of earshot? The answer is simple: because of their medical training. They're taught to make "differential diagnoses"—a process of ruling out various medical possibilities by first imagining the most dangerous diagnoses (brain tumor, aneurysm, meningitis, stroke), then winnowing down the list until only the most likely are left, like garden-variety tension headache.

Playing "rule out" may safeguard against cavalier practitioners who aren't thorough in their detective work. But all too often this Spock-like logic also alienates patients and further fuels their health fears. Doctors forget they're no longer in medical school trying to impress their professors. It's as if they're thinking out loud.

This sort of baffling bedside manner is only one example of how modern medical training keeps doctors from connecting with patients. But it goes to the heart of why so many patients feel let down by conventional medicine. No wonder more and more are seeking healthcare practitioners who work to alleviate their physical problems *and* their emotional worries, rather than add to their anxieties. See Chapter 5 for more on cutting through "doctorese" and improving how you communicate with your physician.

Coaching Patients

In his book *Worried Sick,* Fredric Neuman, M.D., notes that "health anxiety" isn't something to be discouraged or avoided. Rather, it should be viewed as normal.[3] Keys to treating the "worried well," he argues, can't be found in what conventional medicine offers—innumerable tests, procedures, and futile treatments. Nor does "cutting to the chase" work—informing patients bluntly that they're "cranks" and shuttling them off to a psychiatrist or prescribing antidepressants. Rather, Dr. Neuman suggests that health-worriers should inform themselves about all potential ramifications of their condition, real or imagined, and face their fears. And doctors should be there with them, partnering as they explore, instead of turning the other way. (See "Practice Tips for Doctors" on page 39 for respectful ways to discuss alternative therapies with patients.)

Indeed, this may be one of the most important things a doctor can do. Time and again, I've seen that attempts to alleviate vague symptoms with pills and tests alone usually miss the mark. Granted, I don't advocate "enabling" patients with psychological disorders to endlessly search for medical answers (remember my example of the young "worried-well" patient from the previous chapter). But by recognizing that many patients are seeking an emotional and spiritual connection with their practitioner, in addition to relief from their medical woes, doctors can dramatically strengthen the physician-patient bond and significantly improve the care they provide. Indeed, by relentlessly delving into the truth about worrisome problems, then using stress-reduction techniques to attack free-floating anxiety (which is ultimately at the root of all phobias), I've successfully "coached" many patients back to wellness and security.

PRACTICE TIPS FOR DOCTORS:
TALKING TO PATIENTS ABOUT ALTERNATIVES

As more patients turn to complementary and alternative approaches, the need for good information becomes increasingly necessary. Doctors can play a vital role in helping patients sort through various CAM treatments and blend them with mainstream therapies. But they must remain open, be respectful of patients' choices, and be willing to learn more themselves. Here's how:

• **Open communication lines.** Let patients know that your practice is a "safe zone" for discussing CAM healing methods and that you won't be judgmental about their selection of non-conventional approaches. Assure them that you have their best interests at heart and want them to get the best conventional and alternative treatments.

• **Be respectful.** Deriding patients for trying alternatives will only dampen the rapport necessary to ensure that they follow your recommendations. Avoid statements like, "You're not taking any of those supplements, are you?" Or "You're not on one of those crazy fad diets?" To better empathize with patients, imagine yourself proposing an investment scenario to your financial advisor. A skilled advisor may think your scheme is hare-brained, but will patiently guide you to a more rational decision.

• **Avoid derogatory words.** Terms like "quackery" or "placebo" demean patients' intelligence and undermine their sense of personal freedom.

• **Steer clear of categorical statements.** For example, don't say, "St. John's wort *never* works for patients with depression!" Recognize that some claims are controversial, but that conventional medicine also makes controversial claims. Your patients will respect you more for being a compassionate consultant rather than a dictatorial true-believer.

• **Ask questions.** Find out whether patients are seeing other non-traditional practitioners, following special diets, or taking supplements. Make sure your patient questionnaire contains a separate question about the use of nutritional supplements, herbs, and other CAM therapies. Weave it into your normal history-taking about their relationships, sexuality, stress level, and bad health habits.

• **Listen.** The average doctor interrupts patients every ten to fifteen seconds, giving them little chance to air concerns. Take extra time to hear what patients say. Remember that the main reason patients withhold information about unorthodox therapies is because they fear derision or assume mainstream physicians know little about them.

• **Inform yourself.** Take time to read popular magazines to see what they're saying about diet, supplements, herbs, acupuncture, and other natural products or therapies. Then round out your CME (Continuing Medical Education) requirements by attending one of the many fully accredited conferences that are held each year on various aspects of CAM. (See "For Doctors: Getting a CAM Education" on page 46.)

• **Learn about drug-nutrient and drug-herb interactions.** The surest way to gain your patients' confidence is to stay up to date on the potential ramifications of combining CAM therapies with the conventional therapies you're prescribing. (See Resources for Physicians for more on drug-nutrient interactions. Chapters in Part Two also discuss many condition-specific interactions.)

• **Back it up with evidence.** If you think a therapy might be dangerous or worthless, provide your patient with a scientific reference or medical article that supports your view.

• **Talk to patients' alternative practitioners.** By taking time to explore the rationale behind all therapies you may be either pleasantly surprised or remain unconvinced of its value. Either way, you at least learned more and might even develop a network of trusted contacts within the alternative community who can give you the "heads-up" on unfamiliar modalities.

• **NEVER abandon patients.** Don't threaten to drop patients if they pursue a therapy you don't approve of. First of all, it might be considered patient abandonment, resulting in disciplinary action in some jurisdictions. Even worse, it precludes you from monitoring a patient's progress.

TRANSFORMING HEALTH CARE

Where might such a shift in thinking lead medicine? Tel Franklin, M.D., author of *Appreciative Medicine,* envisions a total transformation of the healthcare system that reaches beyond the distinctions of "innovative" versus "orthodox."[4] He writes: "I believe for alternative medicine to be a true alternative, there needs to emerge a new philosophical approach to patient care, a way to redefine health challenges, and an innovative change in the patient–doctor relationship . . . based upon mutual trust, collaboration, and most importantly a 'partnership.'"

As we've seen, efforts in this direction are beginning. One of the more exciting endeavors comes from Johns Hopkins University and American Healthways, a health-risk management company. Late in 2003, more than two hundred patients, physicians, and other medical professionals gathered to talk about what each wants and expects from the other. The resulting consensus report, "Defining the Patient-Physician Relationship for the 21st Century," outlines a few simple recommendations for both patients and doctors that could lead to widespread changes.[5]

Patients should:

• Bring a list of questions to ask the physician. If a friend or family member will be serving as an advocate, make the doctor aware of this, as well.

• Keep a detailed personal medical file, including lab results and prescriptions, and share them with all members of the healthcare team. Make sure the primary physician is kept in the loop regarding appointments with specialists and other providers.

• Assume ultimate responsibility for managing your condition and work with your doctor to set goals and expectations regarding testing, treatment, and self-care practices.

Doctors should:

• Be on time, including scheduled visits and returning patient phone calls.

• Use a social questionnaire for patients to gain a better understanding of non-medical aspects of their lives, including family, education, race, gender, occupation, hobbies, and religious preference.

• Train office staff to provide a friendly and inviting environment.

• Encourage patients to be involved in self-care and offer resources to help them. Work with patients to devise realistic health expectations and goals.

• Be objective when looking at outside information, including non-traditional treatments. Respect patients' views and talk honestly about treatments they feel might be helpful.

"Prospective" Care

An exciting patient-centered approach, called "prospective" care, is also taking hold among health insurers. The aim is to preemptively identify patients who are most likely to develop degenerative conditions, like cardiovascular disease and diabetes, and intervene sooner rather than later (after a condition becomes overly costly to treat). "Prospective" care programs, such as one being pioneered at Duke University, help patients assess their health risks and devise an individualized plan to minimize them.[6] Duke even provides "health coaches" and support groups to help patients carry out their wellness plans.

Granted, this kind of care sounds lavish, and indeed, the additional time spent talking to patients and fashioning a personal health roadmap costs more money (an estimated 1.5 percent more than traditional health plans). Nor are many conventional doctors likely to warm up—at least initially—to the idea of becoming health coaches (a less authoritarian role involving skills more like those used by CAM practitioners). But with 79 percent of healthcare resources currently being expended on the sickest 10 percent of patients, this kind of collaboration is likely to more than pay for itself in the long run.

It is my hope that the future brings more efforts like these—not necessarily to "reinvent the wheel," but to further meld conventional health care with the diet, stress-reduction, lifestyle advice, and partnership approach that CAM practitioners embrace.

BOOSTING MEDICAL LITERACY

What can doctors and patients do now to encourage this melding process and improve their ability to communicate with one another? The first daunting step is to sort through reams of medical information, particularly about CAM approaches. Both physicians and patients need to balance skepticism with openness and achieve a meeting of the minds. Obviously, this is easier said than done.

Admittedly, many CAM approaches haven't yet been rigorously studied, if at all. And the natural-products industry has certainly shot itself in the foot repeatedly by grasping for profits at the price of its own credibility. Dubious claims have sent countless worthless and even dangerous products to the market. But, as we've seen, conventional medicine doesn't have a lock on scientific purity either. Nor is it free of commercial interests.

Interestingly, the Institute of Medicine, an arm of the National Academies that provides independent scientific information on health matters, recently released a lengthy report with wide-ranging recommendations to help consumers and doctors sort through the hodge-podge of nontraditional therapies. It also offered proposals to tighten regulations on herbs and vitamins, boost funding for clinical trials on alternative therapies, and add alternative-medicine courses to medical-school curricula.[7]

In the meantime, how can consumers and their doctors decide about the value—or potential peril—of various medical approaches? I believe the key is to cultivate scientific and medical *literacy*. I've made this my life's work, whether on my daily radio show, in my private practice, in my writings, or when lecturing health professionals and the public.

As the old proverb notes, "Give a man a fish, and he'll eat for a day; teach a man to fish, and he'll eat for life." I believe in not just issuing directives, but also in teaching doctors and patients methods for sifting through the evidence and evaluating it critically.

Making Informed Choices

Another recent report from the Institute of Medicine shows that nearly half of all American adults—90 million people—have trouble understanding and using basic health information, including comprehending a medical form or a doctor's technical instructions about drugs or procedures.[8] In fact, low health literacy, even among well-educated people with strong writing and reading skills, leads to billions of dollars in avoidable healthcare costs, the report noted.

Many in medicine point to this as a sign that full doctor-patient partnerships will never be possible. If patients can't even follow simple written instructions about basic health matters, they argue, how can they be expected to take more responsibility for managing their own chronic conditions or separating CAM wheat from the chafe?

One of CAM's harshest critics, Barry Beyerstein, Ph.D., of Simon Fraser University in British Columbia, epitomizes the view of many physicians:

> Surveys consistently find that, despite our overwhelming dependence on technology, the average citizen of the industrialized world is shockingly ignorant of even the rudiments of science. Consequently, most people lack the knowledge to make an informed choice when they must decide whether a highly touted healthcare product is sensible or not.[9]

While I agree that there's a problem with scientific literacy in this country, I think that attitudes like this are disempowering to patients, and grossly underestimate their capacity to make sensible choices for themselves. Granted, some people are misguided or deluded enough to believe that whatever balm or potion they're reaching for will magically heal them. But countless others are smart consumers—skilled technicians, research scientists, efficient homemakers, teachers, and government officials. They make "scientific" decisions every day. They select cars, plan vacations, evaluate complex political issues before voting, and decide whether to call the pediatrician when their children come down with sore throats. They know themselves and their bodies, but they need help cutting through the thicket of options in the crowded marketplace. See "Educate Yourself" on page 44 for good sources of mainstream and CAM medical information.

Open Dialogue

What physicians and patients need to do is listen to one another without judg-

EDUCATE YOURSELF

Managing your health and partnering with your doctor requires some medical knowledge. The following resources offer reliable studies, links, and articles about both traditional and CAM therapies:

- **National Center for Complementary and Alternative Medicine:** www.nccam.nih.gov/health; (888) 644-6226. A division of the National Institutes of Health. Provides articles and databases.

- **HealthFinder:** www.healthfinder.gov. Consumer-friendly articles, organizations and links from the Department of Health and Human Services.

- **Medline Plus:** www.nlm.nih.gov/medlineplus. A service of the National Library of Medicine and the National Institutes of Health, providing information on over 700 diseases and conditions, lists of hospitals and physicians, a medical encyclopedia and medical dictionary, information on prescription and nonprescription drugs, links to thousands of clinical trials and ability to search for studies on MedLine.

- **PatientInform:** www.patientinform.org/PI/home.jsp. Free online service from leading medical associations providing access to and analysis of up-to-date, reliable research on the diagnosis and treatment of specific diseases.

- **PubMed:** www.ncbi.nlm.nih.gov/entrez/query.fcgi. A service of the National Library of Medicine, which includes public access to MedLine, provides citations for over 15 million studies.

- **PubMed CAM-related articles:** Access www.nlm.nih.gov/nccam/camonpubmed.html and see Resources for Patients for more on where to find medical information.

ment. Stephen Straus, M.D., the Director of the National Center for Complementary and Alternative Medicine (NCCAM), a center of the National Institutes of Health, offers this advice:

> There are times that physicians are afraid their patients will ask them questions about CAM, because they don't know all the answers; and there are many patients who are afraid their physician will think poorly of them. But this is a dialogue that must take place. As a physician, I may not agree with

everything my patient believes in, but it's important that I understand and respect their beliefs. Patients should ask any questions they have about CAM, and physicians should do their best to try to help find good answers and work out a strategy that both should be comfortable with.[10]

For doctors this means remaining open, even if a proposed treatment sounds preposterous (see "For Doctors: Getting a CAM Education" on page 46 for ways that doctors can learn more about alternative medical approaches). Most patients welcome realistic, honest appraisals of the risks and benefits of all treatments they're considering, including CAM therapies. They want a "health coach" rather than a health dictator, one who uses a minimum of scientific jargon and guides them to make smarter, better, health decisions. As the "Practice Tips for Doctors" on page 65 illustrate, the key is courtesy and compassion, particularly for patients who may be suffering from chronic or terminal conditions with few conventional treatment options.

Of course, patients must also be open to their doctor's advice, including the possibility that a conventional approach is the best course of treatment rather than an alternative therapy they'd like to try. Having a doctor they trust—one who is open to both mainstream and CAM approaches and fluent in both—is vital.

Is the Study a Good One?

Part of medical literacy means being able to correctly interpret study results and determine how relevant or significant the findings are. Unfortunately, even doctors don't always get this right. In particular, many conventional physicians believe that complementary and alternative medicine is not evidence-based—that there are few scientific studies supporting its use and most are of poor quality. Yet as we've seen, this isn't always true. Though bad CAM research certainly exists, there are also plenty of good studies. And more are being published all the time. Plus, as noted before, instances of bias and outright fraud also abound in mainstream medical science. Yet most doctors embrace the findings of conventional studies without question.

The key, according to *Lancet* editor Dr. Richard Horton, is for physicians to apply the "precautionary principle."

We [as physicians] must act on facts. . . . and on the most accurate interpretation of them, using the best scientific information. That does not mean we must sit back until we have 100 percent evidence about everything. When the state of the health of people is at stake . . . we should be prepared to take action to diminish those risks even when the scientific knowledge is not conclusive.[11]

If physicians have trouble recognizing legitimate medical claims and interpreting the studies that support them, what's the average citizen to do? I frequently encounter this problem in my office. Not a week goes by that I don't get the heads-up on some promising new herb, supplement, or drug from one of my astute patients. I call them my bird dogs—they retrieve information at an astounding rate, and I welcome their participation.

The problem is, sometimes that information is of high quality, and sometimes it's not. One patient recently revealed that she'd received therapeutic sips of live whipworms for her ulcerative colitis during a trip to Switzerland. As bizarre as it

FOR DOCTORS: GETTING A CAM EDUCATION

The following journals and medical organizations offer valuable CAM information for doctors, including the latest research, as well as educational opportunities.

PROFESSIONAL JOURNALS:

- *Alternative Medicine Alert:* www.ahcpub.com/archive/?efrlk=162. Monthly newsletter providing busy clinicians with evidence-based summaries on alternative and complementary therapies.

- *Alternative Medicine Review:* www.thorne.com/index/mod/amr/a/amr. Peer-reviewed studies and research.

- *Journal of Alternative and Complementary Medicine:* www.liebertpub.com/publication.aspx?pub_id=26. Peer-reviewed studies and research.

MEDICAL CONFERENCE AND EDUCATIONAL PROGRAMS:

- **American Academy of Anti-Aging Medicine (A4M):** www.world-health.net/a4m.html. An international organization of physicians who specialize in therapies designed to extend longevity, including natural HRT and growth hormone.

- **American College for Advancement in Medicine:** www.acam.org or (800) 532-3688. America's oldest organization of physicians prescribing CAM, with a special emphasis on chelation therapy.

- **Institute for Functional Medicine:** www.functionalmedicine.org or (800) 228-0622. An organization of physicians and allied CAM health practitioners trained in nutritional therapies.

See Resources for Physicians for more on CAM education.

sounds, the science was there when I investigated it ("helminthic therapy" was developed at the University of Iowa).[12]

On the other hand, laypersons are often easily bamboozled by pitches for natural nostrums. Many can't distinguish between an infomercial or advertising flyer and a real study. Give them a few high-falutin' scientific words and a couple of diagrams or graphs, and, voilà! They think that's "proof." Indeed, the natural products industry has taken the commercial pitch to high art form.

My suggestions:

• **Consider the source:** If "scientific literature" arrives unsolicited in your mailbox, you may be tempted by its promise to transform your life and health. But consider the possibility that your demographic (over fifty, relatively affluent, a consistent buyer of health products) has placed you on a mailing list that health marketers target.

• **Invoke the TGTBT ("too good to be true") rule:** Many natural products like garlic and fish oil promise almost magical benefits. But beware of exaggerated claims that you'll be rejuvenated, or lose weight effortlessly, or that your sex life will be revolutionized. Nothing can do all that.

Does this mean you should never bring potential products or treatments to your doctor's attention? The answer is no. Your doctor should be receptive. But you should also recognize that he or she is trained to be skeptical. If a treatment is beyond his or her ken, and smacks of "natural" or "alternative," you need to take your best shot by offering the most credible information you can find. That means familiarizing yourself with the difference between "lightweight" evidence and "air-tight."

In a recent article, well-known health author Barry Fox, Ph.D., proposes the following criteria for evaluating studies:[13]

• **Was the study based on a fair premise?** In other words, did researchers stack the deck to prove their conclusions? Examples of studies designed with bias against alternative therapies include a *New England Journal of Medicine* study by cancer researcher Charles Moertel, "proving" that high-dose vitamin C doesn't work in cancer patients.[14] However, he based this conclusion on giving oral vitamin C to end-stage cancer patients who'd already failed to respond to chemo and radiation. Of course, vitamin C didn't work; nothing would! Another study showed that St. John's wort is "ineffective" against depression, but relied on a group of patients so seriously depressed they failed to respond even to conventional antidepressants.[15] Other forms of bias include evaluating natural remedies that can take awhile to work for too short a time—fish oil has "failed" against arthritis in several such studies.

• **Was the appropriate study used?** These days, the "gold standard" for scientific research is the *double-blind, placebo-controlled study*. (In such studies neither researchers nor patients know who is receiving the real treatment or a placebo, so results are less likely to be tainted by preconceived expectations.) This is fine if you're studying drugs, but isn't nearly as useful if you're examining health factors that are more difficult to isolate and measure, like diet or lifestyle.

Epidemiological studies are also popular. But they only point out correlations between a particular diet or lifestyle and its impact on health. In other words, it might be interesting that people in the Balkans often live well past one hundred and consume lots of yogurt containing live cultures. But you can't reasonably infer that lactobacillus is the sole key to their longevity or that sedentary people in America who add yogurt to their fast-food diet will live longer. Unfortunately, the only way to really "prove" that a diet works is by locking people up and carefully measuring and recording all the food they eat—not exactly a practical approach.

Recall studies assess the effects of certain diets by drawing on people's memories of past meals. However, they can be marred by faulty recollections. I personally have trouble remembering what I ate last Thursday, much less in the '70s.

Anecdotal reports also carry their share of problems. Your Aunt Sally may drink fifteen cups of green tea daily for a month and lose twenty pounds. But this needs to be confirmed through more scientific study to establish a plausible *mechanism* for the weight loss that's grounded in biochemistry.

• **Was the data tortured?** Mark Twain once said: "There are lies, damned lies, and statistics." Researchers with an axe to grind have a tendency to apply statistical interpretations to raw data that supports their conclusions. This "observer bias" extends beyond the world of medicine. Witness recent evidence showing that supposedly objective military intelligence was wrong about there being weapons of mass destruction in Iraq.

• **Who funded and conducted the study?** Check your study's pedigree. Not surprisingly, studies supporting the benefits of dietary protein are often underwritten by organizations like the National Livestock and Meat Board; those touting calcium sometimes have support from the dairy industry; and drug studies may be bankrolled by pharmaceutical companies. New full-disclosure rules dictate that any financial ties between researchers and underwriters be fully spelled out. Unfortunately, in the rough-and-tumble—and largely unregulated world—of supplements, such ethical strictures aren't always followed. Stay on the money trail: ask yourself, who will benefit from this scientific conclusion?

- **What do others say about the study?** Do some due diligence. "Google" any study you're about to present to your doctor, and see what recognized medical authorities, both conventional and complementary, are saying about it. But don't get discouraged: Approaches labeled "unscientific," "unproven," or even outright "quackery" by conservative medical groups like the American Heart Association, the Rheumatoid Foundation, or the American Cancer Society tend to enter the mainstream, only years later.

Navigating the Internet

Cyberspace has revolutionized access to medical information. Surveys show that medical searches are among the most popular. As many physicians will attest from the piles of Web printouts that patients bring in, the Internet is where most consumers get their medical information, including news about CAM treatments.

But just as the quality of studies can vary, so can the quality of health websites. To boost medical literacy, doctors and patients also need to learn how to better navigate and analyze the information they find and rule out the extremes. For instance, some medical sites are mere commerce portals dedicated to pushing products with seemingly authoritative claims. Remember the TGTBT rule mentioned earlier.

On the flip side are sites that denounce all CAM therapies. Granted, skepticism is important, but highly critical sites (many pop up on popular search engines like Google or Yahoo) can hardly be considered authorities on CAM. Some, including www.quackwatch.com, apparently have yet to meet a complementary or alternative modality that deserves anything but utter disdain. Even well-established approaches, such as chiropractic, acupuncture, and mind-body techniques, are routinely disparaged.

The following is a set of criteria for "rating" the reliability of health websites, developed by the Health On the Net Foundation (HON), an international non-profit organization of medical experts. About 3,000 websites now meet HON's "Code of Conduct" standards. Look for the HONcode seal on a site's homepage or search for health information among HONcode accredited sites at www.hon.ch/HONcode/Hunt.

When evaluating any site, look for the following "reliability" indicators:

1. **Authority.** All health information on the site is provided by medically trained and qualified professionals—unless clearly stated that advice is from a non-medically qualified individual or organization.

2. **Complementarity.** Information is designed to support, not replace, the relationship that exists between a patient and his or her physician.

3. **Confidentiality.** Data about visitors, including their identity, is respected by

the site. Site owners also honor or exceed the legal requirements of medical/ health information privacy that apply in the country and state where the site is located.

4. **Attribution.** Information on the site is supported by clear references to source data and, where possible, has specific HTML links to that data. The date when a clinical page was last modified is clearly displayed (for example, at the bottom of the page).

5. **Justification.** Any claims about a specific treatment, commercial product, or service are supported by appropriate, balanced evidence in the manner outlined above in Principle 4.

6. **Transparency of authorship.** The site's designers seek to provide the clearest possible information, as well as contact addresses for visitors who want further information or support. The Webmaster displays his/her e-mail address clearly throughout the website.

7. **Transparency of sponsorship.** Support for the site is clearly identified, including the identities of commercial and non-commercial organizations that have contributed funding, services, or material to the site.

8. **Honesty in advertising and editorial policy.** If advertising is a source of funding, it's clearly stated along with a brief description of the site's advertising policy. All advertising and promotional material is clearly distinguishable from the original material created for the site.

Is It "CAM-lite"

Of course, no advice is complete without a few caveats. While the HON guidelines are certainly important for spotting hidden agendas, stodgy adherence to them can also threaten the originality and innovation so integral to the Internet revolution. In other words, just because a health website isn't HONcode accredited doesn't mean it can't provide vital and factual information. After all, it was amateur web "bloggers" who "outed" the phony memo about President Bush's military record during the 2004 presidential campaign. And the first mention of the burgeoning Monica Lewinsky scandal broke on a then-obscure website called the "Drudge Report." Paul Revere, if reincarnated in the twenty-first century, would probably disseminate his message via a non-official "blog."

The point is that the Web democratizes the exchange of information, allowing those with well-founded, sometimes "non-mainstream" messages (but few financial resources or power) to communicate to a mass audience. Thus, you don't have to be a major pharmaceutical corporation, hospital, or government agency anymore to put up a website that offers useful, and sometimes cutting-edge information that may differ from the consensus.

Even so, important scientifically validated health breakthroughs still tend to fall by the wayside without backing from a legitimate accrediting body like HON. Or else, they're only partially accepted, usually in watered-down form. One of my pet peeves is the recent proliferation of what I term "CAM-lite" websites, often sponsored by universities, big hospitals, and government agencies, or posted as subsections of well-established (often HON-accredited) websites. These sites tout themselves as responsible arbiters of all that is evidence-based and reasonable to help consumers sort through the baffling array of CAM modalities. But what is typically offered is a diluted and emasculated version of high-impact CAM therapies.

Don't get me wrong—with so many people hawking snake oil on the Web there's a need for some sort of air-traffic control system. But the therapies that are favorably reviewed on these sites—typically by leading medical authorities (who also tend to be CAM dilettantes)—are mostly innocuous. They don't pose a threat to the prevailing medical paradigm. Typically included are spirituality, meditation, "middle-of the-road" healthy diets, massage techniques, and occasionally acupuncture. However, they're never offered as a substitute for mainstream treatments—but always as an adjunct.

My colleague, Julian Whitaker M.D., recently summed it up in his *Health & Healing* newsletter:

> Conventional medicine has made an attempt to adopt a few CAM therapies. Many hospitals now boast that they provide alternative treatments, and the visualization techniques and acupuncture they offer their patients are certainly beneficial. But do they replace the surgeries and drug therapies that are available in these hospitals? Of course not.
>
> Medical conferences often include a talk or two on one CAM therapy or another, but they are sandwiched between dozens of presentations on the latest drug research. Even conferences that are devoted to CAM therapies give short shrift to hard-hitting, true alternative methods.[16]

While I'm hard-pressed to provide infallible guidelines on how to sort "CAM" from "CAM-lite," I suggest that, at the very least, savvy web-surfers compare sites to get a balanced view of controversial therapies.

Remember, too, that no website (CAM, CAM-lite, or otherwise) is a substitute for first-hand research. If studies about a particular therapy are available, go directly there rather than take a hand-me-down claim—positive or negative—at face value. PubMed, a service of the National Library of Medicine, provides citations for over 15 million studies, including CAM-only, peer-reviewed articles. See "Educate Yourself" on page 44 and Resources for Patients in the back of the book for more helpful websites.

The more you familiarize yourself with available medical information, the better you'll be able to talk to your doctor in a language he or she understands. And the more likely you'll be to receive the care you seek. All are important pieces of the "integrative" medical vision I've outlined here.

In Part Two, we'll take this vision a step further by exploring how healthy patients can work with their doctor to head off disease and stay healthy. We'll also examine how those with specific medical conditions, like heart disease and cancer, can collaborate with their physicians to find the best conventional and alternative treatments available and devise a customized holistic healing approach that's right for them.

PART TWO

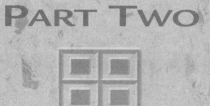

Making Knowledgeable Decisions, Getting the Care You Want

Getting a Real Physical Exam

The superior physician helps before the early budding of the disease . . .
The inferior physician begins to help when the disease has already developed.

—FROM *THE YELLOW EMPEROR'S CLASSIC OF INTERNAL MEDICINE*

One of the most hallowed rituals of modern medicine is "The Physical," a tradition that is re-enacted annually by millions of conscientious Americans. We sit on cold examination tables in ill-fitting paper gowns waiting to be poked and probed, allowing our bodily fluids to be sampled and analyzed—all in the belief that fulfilling this yearly rite will safeguard our continued health and longevity.

But, according to a recent *New York Times* article, our implicit faith in this exam may be misplaced. Indeed, checkups for people with no medical complaint—the single biggest reason for visiting a doctor—may be nothing more than an empty annual observance, providing little useful information about an individual's actual health. As the article notes:

> . . . . In a series of reports that began in 1989 and is still continuing, an expert committee sponsored by the federal Agency for Healthcare Research and Quality, an arm of the Department of Health and Human Services, found little support for many of the tests commonly included in a typical physical exam for symptomless people.
>
> It found no evidence, for example, that routine pelvic, rectal and testicular exams made any difference in overall survival rates for those with no symptoms of illness.
>
> It warned that such tests can lead to false alarms, necessitating a round of expensive and sometimes risky follow-up tests. And even many tests that are useful, like cholesterol and blood pressure checks, need not be done every year . . .[1]

In this chapter we'll look at why conventional medicine continues to push patients to get "ineffectual" yearly checkups. Plus, we'll examine ways to boost the predictive value of a physical exam, including tests ignored by most of mainstream medicine. Not only can these tests provide a meaningful glimpse into the body's overall health, but they may also detect early signs of future medical problems.

TESTING 1, 2, 3 . . .

"Evidence-based" medicine is the new buzzword these days. The aim is to craft recommendations for when to use particular tests and other medical procedures, based on scientific evidence about what actually works and what doesn't. Toward that end, medical scientists have begun subjecting many venerated medical tests to the harsh light of experimental validation—and have found several lacking.

Indeed, certain tests are actually without any clinical basis whatsoever. Case in point: hundreds of thousands of women annually receive Pap smears to detect cervical cancer after having undergone a hysterectomy—an operation that surgically removes all traces of the cervix! Even after a U.S. Government Task Force noted the inconsistency and devised physician guidelines encouraging them to cease giving Pap smears to women with hysterectomies, there's been absolutely no reduction in the number of such unnecessary procedures performed![2]

Other tests that haven't passed "evidence-based" muster include routine chest x-rays for people without respiratory symptoms, screening ECGs (electrocardiograms) for those without signs of heart trouble, and fecal occult blood tests (FOBT) for detecting blood in the stool (a possible indicator of colon cancer).

Even the venerable PSA (prostate specific antigen) test for prostate cancer has recently come under fire for its high rates of false positives and false negatives, and because studies show that, while more prostate cancers are found early with it, there's no real boost in quality of life or longevity. Likewise, medical authorities have largely abandoned their appeals for women to perform monthly breast exams because the practice hasn't boosted the rate of discovery of breast cancer or survival from the disease.

All this bespeaks a health system in flux. As noted before, use of many tests may be little more than hollow annual traditions, performed simply because doctors were once taught to do them and patients have come to expect them. Worse, the threat of malpractice litigation may reinforce reliance on tests whose value is at best marginal. And a few may be performed simply because doctors and hospitals profit from them. Providing annual physicals is a big business for the healthcare industry, adding up to about $7 billion per year!

Limitations of "Usual and Customary"

A typical physical for men and women over age fifty usually consists of a tip-to-toe inspection. Blood pressure is measured. Then blood is drawn for a "SMAC" test (which monitors several bodily functions, including liver and kidney function) and a "CBC," or complete blood count, which determines whether anemia, blood diseases or infection are present. "Sed" (sedimentation) rate is also measured, indicating the presence of inflammation somewhere in the body (though it's not sensitive enough for the kind of inflammation that could lead to early heart disease or cancer). The physical may also include a "lipid profile," which has become increasingly popular now that cholesterol-lowering drugs are available. Never mind that fully one-third of fatal heart attacks occur in individuals with "normal" values.

Clearly, this traditional exam is missing a lot. Lately, health-conscious, aging baby boomers have begun clamoring for more comprehensive testing. As a result, costly "executive" health-screening programs are proliferating. Upscale enclaves like Newport Beach, Scottsdale, and Fort Lauderdale have seen a boom in diagnostic centers that offer "whole body scans" to forecast disease.

I've seen this trend in my own practice. Recently, a wealthy prospective patient from an oil-rich Middle Eastern country (with no specific physical problems) contacted the Hoffman Center for information about a wellness exam and workup. His assistants arranged the visit and asked about the tests we intended to perform. When my staff replied that this would depend on what his medical history revealed, they said we needn't bother with the history, that price was no object. The patient wanted every single test we offered!

I had to laugh when I thought about the hundreds of different scans, breathing tests, exercise tests, blood tests, saliva tests, even sleep tests we provide. I resisted exploiting his wealth and naiveté and informed him that we'd only order tests directed at his specific issues.

To Test or Not to Test

The reason involves a simple statistical quirk, unknown to most laypersons, that makes such all-out testing impractical and unwise. For one thing, the more you test for unlikely diagnoses, the more false positives you encounter. So if a neurotic patient, for example, were to demand an HIV test after every safe sex encounter (just to be sure!), the chances of finding a falsely elevated test score, rare as that might be, would be infinitely higher than the likelihood of spotting a true HIV infection. The risk is compounded with less reliable tests, like full body scans. More often than not, what they reveal are disconcerting but harmless shadows and anomalies (humorously dubbed "incidentalomas" by some doctors) rather than real problems. Even "routine" stress tests, x-rays, and ECGs sometimes fall prey to this statistical principle, and subject otherwise healthy individuals with no heightened risks or complaints to unnecessary anguish.

As you collaborate with your doctor on reasonable testing goals, consider this as well: a decision to test is often a decision to treat. In other words, once you've crossed the line of awareness with a positive test result, you can no longer ignore its consequences. For example, we now have the ability to test for the BRCA 1 and 2 oncogenes, which predispose women to breast cancer. Women who test positive for these genes, especially those with primary relatives who develop cancer at early ages, sometimes feel compelled to undergo "prophylactic" bilateral mastectomies and even hysterectomies (because of associated higher risk of ovarian cancer). They may never develop cancer, but once a woman chooses to undergo the test she must be prepared to act on bad news. Otherwise it becomes "too much information." Remember, one person's need-to-know can be another's medical nightmare.

Yet another consideration is whether insurers will pay for tests. Many conventional doctors hew carefully to insurers' reimbursement schedules when deciding

GETTING YOUR INSURER TO PAY

When your insurance company says "no" to a medical test or other care you seek, following a few simple steps may help you get the decision reversed in your favor. Here are a few critical points from Drs. Jason Theodosakis and David T. Feinberg (authors of *Don't Let Your HMO Kill You*):[3]

1. **Don't get angry**—but do get involved. Insurance companies want to keep costs down, and that means denying payment for care and medications that they feel are not positively necessary. Don't take this personally. A denial-of-care notice is often just a simple business decision made by a computer or after a cursory review by insurance-company employees.

2. **Hold on to written records**—not just the denial-of-care notice but all correspondence from the insurance company, in the event that your case escalates over time and eventually is heard by a panel of reviewers.

3. **Do some research.** Many medical organizations have set up "practice guidelines"—suggested standards for basic care—which you will find on their websites. For instance, if coverage is denied for a test that's been shown to accurately predict heart disease, you could use this fact to further your case. (There are various websites. See www.americanheart.org, for example, and type "practice guidelines" in the search box.)

4. **Call your insurance company** and say, "I am appealing my denied care." Then put it in writing with a traceable letter sent by certified or registered

on tests for their patients. This is in keen contrast to complementary physicians, whose preferred tests are often deemed "not medically necessary" by insurers. While I like to save patients money, I think that too strict adherence to standard testing guidelines shortchanges them from getting the best workup possible. Besides, as the list below indicates, "unconventional" tests often leap from insurance limbo to the mainstream when enough doctors and patients advocate for them. I'm proud to say I championed use of these now widely employed tests (discussed in greater detail later in this chapter) back when they were considered "unnecessary":

- **DEXA scan:** Checks bone density for early warning of osteoporosis
- **EBT heart scan:** Finds early calcification in coronary arteries

mail, overnight delivery, or fax. Make sure to keep all receipts for your records. Then, have faith. Studies show that about 50 percent of the cases that go to neutral outside panels are decided in favor of the patient.

5. **Notify your department of human resources.** Send a copy of your letter to the head of personnel or human resources (HR) at work. Since this department actually purchases medical and other insurance on your behalf, the insurance company sees it, not you, as the customer. When the HR department puts pressure on the insurance company, things happen.

6. **If you think a test or treatment is urgent or required, get it.** Launch an appeal later, when you have less to lose. Trying to save a few dollars by delaying care is never worth the risk to your health.

7. **Finally, let your doctor help.** Enlisting a doctor's help in the appeals process can make a big difference in your case. Doctors are used to dealing with insurance companies, and they know the lingo. That's why it's a good idea to cultivate positive relationships with your healthcare providers. Ask your physician to:

- Write a letter of "medical necessity" about the test or treatment in question to submit to the insurance company.
- Speak with one of the nurse reviewers or medical directors who is reviewing your case for the insurance company.

8. **Visit Dr. Theodosakis's website:** www.drtheo.com to download forms that will assist you in writing letters of appeal.

- **Gluten profile:** Provides evidence of underlying celiac disease

- **HDL cholesterol test:** Looks for too-low levels of this "good" heart-healthy cholesterol

- **High-sensitivity C-reactive protein test:** Detects inflammation of blood vessels leading to heart attacks

- **Homocysteine test:** Detects elevated levels of this amino acid—a risk factor for blood clots, strokes, and heart attacks

Certainly, other tests considered "cutting-edge" today will likely become *de rigueur* in the future. In the meantime, you and your doctor can help convince insurers to pay for non-mainstream tests using strategies offered by Drs. Jason Theodosakis and David T. Feinberg, authors of *Don't Let Your HMO Kill You*.[4] See "Getting Your Insurer to Pay" on page 58.

BEEFING UP THE TRADITIONAL PHYSICAL

I think it's no coincidence that well-educated baby boomers are leading the charge for better health information. They're literate, informed, and as part of the "Sputnik Generation," they're grade-crazy. To some, this may seem neurotic and narcissistic, but I think this trait makes them champion patients. What they want is a full status report on their health, not a hasty glance that overlooks important pieces. The physical exam I'm about to describe, including the tests I recommend, goes well beyond the general health snapshot of conventional physicals. Not only can it help pinpoint life-threatening diseases, but it also provides a "report card" so patients can better fend off degenerative conditions and preserve optimal health. What it doesn't do is merely add worry and uncertainty.

Taking a Closer Look

From a complementary medicine standpoint, "beefing up" the traditional physical exam often means starting with a patient's appearance. Inviting your doctor in for a closer look can yield important clues to possible underlying health problems. Many of them are easily treated via diet change, supplements, and exercise. And, if noted early enough, can even be averted before they mushroom into more serious conditions. Getting the once-over on your general appearance also allows you and your doctor to chart out which additional tests might be required ("Practice Tips" on page 65 helps doctors work with patients who want non-standard tests). We'll discuss some of these later in this chapter.

Skin, Hair, and Nails

Often there's a disconnect between a patient's chronological age and biological age—some look older than their actual age and some look younger. Part of it is programmed genetically, and part is due to environmental factors. Skin suppleness, tone, and the presence of wrinkles—all superficial hallmarks of aging—provide important hints about how the rest of the body is aging.

One thing I note during physicals is how "glycosylated" a patient looks. Think Keith Richards of Rolling Stones rock fame, whose reptilian skin makes him a poster boy for glycosylation. This aging process (analogous to the searing of meat or the browning of bread) occurs when free radicals cause sugars and proteins to bond. It's accelerated in people who smoke or have excess sun exposure, especially if they also have high blood sugar.

A doctor can also glean important clues about how fast harmful internal degenerative processes are ravaging the body by noting the rate at which skin collagen loses its elasticity, giving it a mottled, crepey appearance. Strategies for slowing the onslaught include controlling blood sugar, eliminating harmful pro-oxidants like smoking, excess sun, and chemicalized food, and recommending specific dietary and supplemental antioxidants. For more on this, read Dr. Nicholas Perricone's book *The Wrinkle Cure.*

Certain other skin changes including an excess of skin tags, or dark patches of skin on the back, neck, or under the arms (*Acanthosis nigricans*), are also predictive of blood sugar abnormalities, such as Syndrome X and diabetes (see next under "Waist and Hips").

In addition, paradoxically, both skin that is excessively oily or skin that is dry and flaky can be signs of essential fatty acid deficiencies. Likewise, hair that is overly greasy, prone to dandruff, or dry, lusterless and unruly, can also indicate deficiencies of good oils and fats in the diet.

In addition, doctors should keep an eye out for physical signs of low thyroid function, including thinning hair, dry skin, and fragile nails. All are important clinical signs of possible of hypothyroidism—especially if someone also has palpable thyroid nodules, swollen facial features (a sign of abnormal water retention), sluggish reflexes, or weight gain.

Nail color, texture, and strength also offer a glimpse into a patient's overall nutritional status and health. For instance, nails that are susceptible to fungal infections may indicate a breech in the patient's immune defenses, or a diet so high in refined carbohydrates that it fosters growth of sugar-loving fungi.

Waist and Hips

Another evaluation frequently skipped by conventional doctors is what I like to call the "$1.98 Insulin Resistance Test." If your doctor took a few seconds to wrap one of those inexpensive cloth tape measures used by seamstresses around your waist, then around your hips, it could yield a helpful benchmark called the "waist-to-hip ratio." You can calculate it yourself by dividing your waist measurement by your hip measurement.

In men, if the ratio is greater than 1.0, there is a strong likelihood of insulin resistance or metabolic syndrome (also called Syndrome X). In women, who naturally have wider hips, a ratio of greater than 0.75 may indicate emerging problems. Insulin resistance is a reduced sensitivity in the tissues to the action of insulin, which causes the body to overcompensate by producing more insulin. This can lead to a cluster of abnormalities, including high blood pressure, central obesity, and abnormal triglyceride and cholesterol levels. Taken together, these factors can mean a heightened risk of heart disease, diabetes, and stroke. See Chapter 6 on heart disease for more about preventing and treating Syndrome X.

Muscles

Muscle tone and size can be an important health parameter, not just a vanity issue. Loss of muscle volume proceeds at about 10 percent per decade after age forty. Therefore, resistance exercise that maintains and builds muscle is an important hedge against the degenerative processes of aging.

Lack of muscle tone in men, along with a soft, protuberant abdomen or sagging breast tissue (gynecomastia) can also be tip-offs to a low testosterone state, often confirmed with blood testing. For treatments, see the section on andropause in Chapter 10.

Mouth and Cheeks

Because people with periodontal disease are more likely to have inflammatory changes in their arterial walls leading to premature blockage, gums can furnish important clues to heart disease risk. Additionally, the presence of numerous silver fillings can boost risk of increased toxic body burdens of mercury, something we'll discuss later in this chapter.

See if you can also get your doctor to tap your cheek lightly with a reflex hammer to elicit a "Chvostek's reflex," an involuntary lip twitch that often indicates a hidden magnesium deficiency.

Blood Pressure

Most doctors check blood pressure (BP) while patients are either sitting or lying on the exam table. However, I recommend a more comprehensive check, which involves measuring BP while someone shifts positions from lying or sitting to standing. For most people, blood pressure holds steady with only a modest increase in heart rate during such a shift. But patients with distressed regulation of their involuntary nerve functions will actually see their blood pressure drop while their heart rate soars. These patients are likely to have problems with fatigue, insomnia, anxiety, irritable bowel syndrome, headaches, or dizziness, which can be halted by drinking more fluids, replacing minerals via supplementation, or taking herbs that support adrenal function. Occasionally, beta blockers must be prescribed to tame adrenaline surges and block rapid heart rate.

Breathing

During a quiet moment, your doctor should also examine your breathing—something a surprising number of patients don't do correctly. The ideal involves smooth, gradual expansion of the abdomen while the chest remains relatively quiet, akin to relaxed yoga breathing. Shallow chest breathers lock their abdominal muscles. At the same time, receptors in the chest wall feed back distress signals to the brain, resulting in chronic anxiety, panic attacks, and overproduction of stress hormones.

Heart

Listening to the heart has become a bit of a lost art. Noisy offices and rushed exams make it harder to perform, but also young doctors are now more reliant on high-tech evaluations, like echocardiograms, to spot heart valve problems. In the old days, ace cardiologists could pretty reliably locate and diagnose valve problems by re-positioning patients and having them hold their breath or exhale while listening carefully with the stethoscope. The point is that one of the most common heart valve abnormalities, mitral valve prolapse (MVP), is frequently missed in conventional exams.

While not considered a dangerous condition—typically requiring only a few precautionary measures, like prophylactic antibiotics before dental procedures—MVP can nonetheless explain a host of medical woes, like shortness of breath and panic attacks. For more on treating MVP, read my book *Natural Therapies for Mitral Valve Prolapse* (see Resources for Patients).

More "Free" Physical Tests

Often the simplest observances have the greatest prognostic value. For example, the inability to stand up unassisted from a sitting position actually predicts a higher risk of mortality. More exercise and strength training is indicated in these cases. Likewise, the speed at which your pulse normalizes after exertion is also a reliable test of cardiovascular conditioning. A slower response means poorer heart function and a need for more life-extending physical activity. In addition, higher systolic blood pressure (the upper number in the BP reading) shortly after exercise often indicates an elevated risk for heart attacks, particularly in middle-aged men.[5]

TESTING FOR TOXICITY

One downside of modern life is that nearly every product, from house paint to dish detergents, is awash in synthetic chemicals and environmental toxins. Unfortunately, conventional physicians often fail to alert patients to the physical harm that may result from eating, drinking, touching, or breathing these toxins long-term. There is increasing awareness, for instance, that lead, mercury, cadmium, and organic chemicals from pollution and many household products play a role in ailments, including hypertension, Alzheimer's disease, cognitive impairment, and kidney disease. In addition, "endocrine-disruptors" found in common household products like plastics (which mimic natural hormones) have been shown to wreak hormonal havoc in the body, affecting the breasts, uterus, prostate, and brain.

In one recent "body burden" study led by the Mount Sinai School of Medicine, the Environmental Working Group, and Commonweal, researchers found an average of 91 industrial compounds, pollutants, and other chemicals in the urine and blood of nine volunteers (none of them worked with chemicals on the job or lived near an industrial facility).[6] A total of 167 chemicals were detected in the group—76 known carcinogens in humans or animals, 94 toxic to the brain and nervous system, and 79 implicated in birth defects.

A more comprehensive study by the U.S. Centers for Disease Control measured 116 toxic compounds in the bodies of volunteers, including chlorinated solvents, pesticides, PCBs (polychlorinated biphenyls), and heavy metals, like lead and mercury.[7]

Body Burden Testing

Because standard blood tests reveal only very high levels of toxic metals in the blood and do not measure how much is stored in tissues, I recommend a "provocative chelation" test, during which patients are given a pill several times a week, called DMSA (dimercaptosuccinic acid). This "oral chelator" grabs on to toxic metals and ushers them safely out of the body. The process is then followed up with a morning urine collection that's sent to a lab for analysis.

Though controversial, I believe this test provides a better reflection of body-burden toxics. And because exposure to health-damaging compounds is so pervasive, I make this test available to any patient who requests it so they can devise an action plan to minimize exposures and, if necessary, begin detoxification. (See "Beyond Conventional Tests" on page 70 for tips on requesting "non-standard" tests.)

Unfortunately, testing for the thousands of other non-metal environmental pollutants that contaminate our water, air, and food presents a far greater chal-

PRACTICE TIPS FOR DOCTORS: WHEN PATIENTS WANT MORE TESTS

• **Listen** to their reasons for seeking additional tests and keep an open mind.

• **Attend** a complementary medicine conference (see Resources for Physicians). Listen to lectures, talk to attendees, and visit the booths to find out about the latest advancements in "complementary diagnostics."

• **Understand** that the rationale for testing in complementary medicine might be more preventive than strictly diagnostic. Remember, too, that cholesterol testing and bone density tests were once experimental and their use for screening controversial. Now they've moved to the forefront of detection. Even if a test isn't crucial for clinching a traditional diagnosis, if it will point the way toward healthful behaviors in your patient, consider ordering it.

lenge. Some states don't permit doctors to assess patients' bodily chemical burden because controversy rages over how much is too much. Check with your doctor about whether these tests are available where you live. For more on the health impact of toxic exposures, check out my book *Intelligent Medicine*. See Resources for Patients to learn about environmental medicine, which explores the link between disease and environmental toxins.

Testing Labs

Ask your doctor to check out the extensive menu of tests available from the following labs:

• **Doctor's Data, Inc:** www.doctorsdata.com. Provides data on levels of toxic and essential elements in hair, and elements, amino acids, and metabolites in blood and urine; (800) 323-2784.

• **Immunosciences Lab, Inc.:** www.immuno-sci-lab.com/index2.html. Develops esoteric tests and helps clinicians diagnose very complex immune system diseases; (800) 950-4686.

• **Metametrix Clinical Laboratory:** www.metametrix.com. Offers a full range of tests, including metabolic profiles, hormone profiles, and oxidative stress indicators; (800) 221-4640.

More testing labs are listed in Resources for Patients.

OTHER USEFUL TESTS

In addition to the standard preventive tests offered during a conventional physical, you and your doctor should work together to determine which of the following tests make sense for you and how often to get them. (For a list of routine tests, including Pap smears and blood pressure checks, recommended during a standard physical, consult guidelines like Park Nicollet Health Advisor's Check-up Schedule. See Resources for Patients for specific recommendations.)

As you decide on additional tests beyond the norm, keep in mind any physical symptoms or complaints you may be experiencing, as well as diet, lifestyle, and stress factors that could provide clues to potential problem areas. Lab Tests Online (http://labtestsonline.org/site/index.html) lists hundreds of lab test descriptions and recommendations for specific conditions. (To help you prioritize if money is an issue, see "When You Can't Afford a Mega-Workup" below.) These higher priority tests are indicated in the next section with asterisks behind them.

Fitness and Metabolism

The following tests go beyond traditional measures of overweight and sugar metab-

---

WHEN YOU CAN'T AFFORD A MEGA-WORKUP

The cost of medical tests can really add up. If your insurer won't pay for all the tests I've described in this chapter and you can't afford them yourself, consider opting for my Top Ten. These tests—along with the SMAC, CBC, a urinalysis, lipid profile, and thyroid function test (all standard in most physicals)—can make a real difference in helping you maintain optimum health.

1. **Body Composition Analysis** (now available at most gyms)
2. **DHEA**
3. **Essential Fatty Acid Profile**
4. **Ferritin**
5. **Glucose Tolerance**
6. **Hemoglobin A1c**
7. **High-Sensitivity C-Reactive Protein**
8. **Homocysteine**
9. **Vitamin B$_{12}$**
10. **Vitamin D**

olism to more effectively pinpoint your underlying risk for major diseases, such as cancer and heart disease:

Body Composition Analysis*

Simply measuring a patient's height and weight doesn't cut it anymore. The National Heart Lung and Blood Institute, which convened in 1998 to revise its guidelines on what constitutes overweight, redefined it as a body mass index, or BMI, of greater than 25 (the cutoff for obesity is 30 or greater). The BMI is a complex calculation relating weight to body surface area. (Calculate your BMI at http://nhlbisupport.com/bmi/bmicalc.htm.)

Instantaneously, 37 million heretofore-normal Americans (65 percent) were propelled into the ranks of the overweight. That includes President Bush, who, at 6 feet and 194 pounds, with a BMI of 26.4, falls into the overweight category. Even yours truly—an inveterate runner, swimmer, bicyclist, and weight lifter, 5'10" and 178 pounds—clocks in with an over-the-limit BMI of 25.5. What's wrong with this picture?

Since muscle is heavier than fat, BMI overestimates risk in athletic individuals with muscular physiques, and underestimates it in seemingly thinner, older, or out-of-shape individuals who carry concealed flab.

Enter a new technology, called impedance plethysmography. While subject to some imprecision (especially the consumer versions for home use), the technique involves sending painless electrical currents through the body to measure the percentage of fat vs. lean muscle and tissue, an important early warning for excess body fat accumulation that more effectively predicts cardiovascular disease and cancer risk than weight alone. Plus, it can help doctors and their overweight patients formulate more realistic weight loss goals. Interestingly, when exercise is teamed with an appropriate diet, and supported by vitamins, supplements, and hormonal support with DHEA and/or testosterone (see below under "Hormonal Balance"), body composition often improves with or without dramatic weight changes. Even someone who loses a "mere" ten pounds can completely turn their health around if they have replaced fifteen pounds of fat with five pounds of new muscle—often dubbed the "My Clothes Fit Better!" syndrome.

Glucose Tolerance Test*

Testing for blood sugar the old way—a fasting test performed as part of the SMAC analysis—can miss the vast majority of patients with abnormal glucose metabolism, which often leads to diabetes and heart disease.

In its place, I recommend the oral glucose tolerance test (GTT), a dynamic blood test that I've used for twenty years to measure patients' response to a sugar challenge. The GTT helps to more precisely diagnose individuals with multiple unexplained symptoms (including fatigue, anxiety, palpitations, hot flashes, even seizures) who may be suffering from unpredictable dips of blood sugar, commonly known as hypoglycemia. The test also better detects spikes of insulin that appear after eating carbohydrates (a possible sign of Syndrome X) than traditional fasting tests.

Circulatory Assessment

Standard blood pressure and cholesterol tests often uncover heart disease after it's already well along. The following tests help detect earlier, subtler signs—such as beginning plaque buildup and arterial inflammation—before they develop into full-blown heart disease:

Comprehensive Cardio Panel

The presence of artery-clogging LDL (low-density lipoprotein) cholesterol is often the major focus of conventional cardiovascular exams. But multiple risk factors, including inflammation within the bloodstream, also contribute to heart disease. I recommend the following additional cardio tests, particularly for men after age thirty-five and women after forty (though children as young as seven sometimes show evidence of plaque buildup and arterial stiffening). In addition, patients with hypertension, obesity, a strong family history of heart disease, and a sedentary lifestyle should also get them. These tests allow me to target specific risk factors, like arterial blockages, that can be treated (usually with lifestyle interventions) or even reversed. See Chapter 6 for more on preventing and treating heart disease.

High-Sensitivity C-Reactive Protein Test*: This test measures levels of C-reactive protein in the blood, a substance produced by the liver in response to inflammation in the blood vessels. For women, in particular, a heightened level of C-reactive protein is an important sign of susceptibility to heart attack and stroke.

Fibrinogen: This blood test predicts "stickiness" of blood platelets. Elevated levels are believed to play a role in clogging arteries (atherosclerosis), a principal piece of the heart disease puzzle.

Homocysteine*: When elevated, this amino acid may irritate blood vessels, leading to blockages and clots. A simple blood test detects excess amounts, which can be corrected with proper diet and supplements, including folic acid, although recent studies cast doubt on whether nutritional support with B vitamins can actually reduce risk of heart attack and stroke (see "Revisiting Controversies" on page 109).

Lipoprotein (a) or Lp(a): Particles that transport cholesterol in the blood. Doctors typically focus on "good" high-density lipoproteins and "bad" low-density lipoproteins, but fail to test for elevated levels of this less familiar type (a key inherited risk factor in cardiovascular disease).

Hemoglobin A1c*: Hemoglobin A1c forms as sugar in the blood attaches to hemoglobin in the red blood cells. Traditionally, the hemoglobin A1c blood test was used only as a "report card" to help diabetics measure their average blood glucose (sugar) level over time. The higher the blood sugar, the more hemoglobin A1c. Researchers now believe that elevated hemoglobin A1c levels (even marginal elevations) may also be a prime risk factor for heart disease and also directly reflect the body's level of harmful glycosylation.

Carotid Doppler Test

This is a simple relatively inexpensive and totally non-invasive ultrasound test of blood vessels in the neck, which can provide an early "heads-up" about plaque development in the arteries leading to the brain. With the carotid Doppler test we no longer have to wait for strokes or TIAs (transient ischemic attacks or "mini strokes") to determine whether arterial blockages are beginning.

EBT (Electron Beam Tomography)

Initially treated with skepticism, this heart scan can help pinpoint who is at high risk for heart disease by assessing the amount of calcium around the coronary arteries. (The more calcium deposits, usually the greater the degree of heart disease.)

The EBT scan is best used as a "tie-breaker" for patients at intermediate risk. Those who've had angina or heart attacks can probably safely bypass it because they will undergo aggressive treatment anyway, as can very young patients with highly favorable lipid profiles. Medium-risk patients, however, are often reassured when an EBT test reveals minimal or no plaque. Likewise, young patients with only slightly raised cholesterol often discover dangerously high plaque scores and can intervene early with aggressive diet, lifestyle, and statin treatments. If left untreated plaque usually increases by about 20 percent per year.

Nutritional Status

Many vitamin and nutritional deficiencies can lead to poor health and disease. Catching deficiencies early with the following tests and implementing targeted dietary changes and nutritional supplementation may help avert potential health problems:

Vitamin D*

I find it remarkable that most physicians will prescribe powerful drugs like Fosamax and Actonel at the drop of a hat to prevent osteoporosis (bone loss) without even considering whether patients have adequate levels of vitamin D. This vitamin, along with calcium, is absolutely essential for bone health.

Research now shows that a high percentage of women are deficient in vita-

BEYOND CONVENTIONAL TESTS

During a recent visit to her doctor, Elaine Santos, a forty-three-year-old college librarian, learned that her cholesterol was slightly elevated. Her doctor told her not to worry and suggested that she cut down on high-cholesterol foods and consider a statin drug.

While searching online one evening, Elaine read about EBT (electron beam tomography), a cutting-edge heart scan that allows patients—even those with minimal risk factors—to assess the level of calcium and plaque accumulations in their coronary arteries. Though controversial, Elaine decided to ask her doctor to order one for her. The following is part of their exchange:

Elaine: Dr. Melvin, I just want to be sure I'm not headed for major heart problems. I brought in some literature about the EBT and am hoping you'll agree I should get one.

Dr. Melvin: Whoa . . . your cholesterol is only a little high and you don't have any other risk factors. I can prescribe a statin drug if you're really worried, but I don't think the EBT is going to tell us much more than we already know. Frankly, most doctors are still skeptical about it.

Elaine: But regular tests for heart disease don't always detect problems until it's too late. There may be other things I can do now to prevent problems later on.

Dr. Melvin: I really think you're overreacting. Let's just try the statin and see what happens.

Elaine: Will you at least look at my literature before you decide anything?

Dr. Melvin: (sighs) When I get a chance . . . in the meantime here's a prescription to get you started.

Elaine: I'm sorry, Dr. Melvin. I know we've been together a long time, but maybe I should see another doctor who's more willing to consider my thoughts.

Occasionally, it's necessary to "fire" a doctor who doesn't take your feelings and input seriously. Elaine ultimately found another physician who ordered the EBT scan. She was relieved when no evidence of plaque buildup was found. But she knew that even a zero score doesn't guarantee that arteries are "bullet-proof." With her doctor's help, she embarked on a preventive regimen, including a heart-healthy diet, daily exercise, and supplement program, which ultimately lowered her cholesterol to safe levels without statins.

min D, and current dietary recommendations are shortchanging them. At particular risk are those living in northern latitudes where sunlight is inadequate from November to March (the skin produces vitamin D in response to sun exposure). Additionally, our current paranoia about skin cancer is causing many fearful individuals to either swath themselves in SPF creams or avoid the sun altogether.

Other maladies linked to vitamin D deficiency include: rheumatoid arthritis, multiple sclerosis, psoriasis, unexplained body aches, muscle weakness, insulin resistance, diabetes, depression, and even colon and prostate cancer.

Folic Acid

This critical B vitamin may be a key protective factor against cardiovascular disease and some cancers, although the value of B vitamins supplementation for cardiovascular prevention remains controversial. Folic acid deficiency (detected via a blood test) raises homocysteine levels. Folic acid may also play a supporting role in treatment of arthritis, fibromyalgia, fatigue, and depression, probably by recharging levels of S-adenosyl methionine (Sam-e). This naturally occurring chemical boosts synthesis of key neurotransmitters and supports detoxification.

Vitamin B_{12}*

Deficiency of this vital energy vitamin is far more common than typically recognized, particularly among vegetarians and individuals whose bodies can't adequately absorb it. B_{12} deficiency is implicated in fatigue, depression, peripheral neuropathy, and many unexplained neurological conditions—even some cases of dementia and other cognitive or memory problems.

Ferritin*

Though not typically performed as part of the standard SMAC, or basic blood chemistry test, this iron test is nonetheless extremely useful. Even when patients aren't suffering from obvious anemia, the ferritin test can reveal subtle iron deficiency—a particular problem for vegetarians, children, and young women. Iron deficiency can impair memory and cognition, result in a fatigued, dragged-out feeling, worsen learning disabilities, lead to poor immunity, and recently has been implicated in restless leg syndrome. Indeed, low iron can literally erode your IQ, and may be responsible for a significant percentage of childhood attention deficit disorder (ADD), especially in young girls.

On the other hand, excess levels of ferritin may reveal a common, treatable genetic tendency toward iron overload, called hemochromatosis, which can damage the liver, accelerate atherosclerosis, and even predispose individuals to Alzheimer's disease and Parkinson's disease. Treatment involves restricting iron intake and sometimes giving blood.

Ionized Calcium and Magnesium

This sophisticated blood test reveals an individual's "available balance" of these key minerals. Other conventional tests for calcium and magnesium are less sensitive in picking up suboptimal levels. Magnesium deficiency is associated with panic disorders and agoraphobia, migraine headaches, muscle spasms, back and neck pain, fibromyalgia, fatigue, PMS, hypertension, and heart disease. Inadequate calcium intake and absorption results in low bone density. Too high calcium levels can lead to hyperparathyroidism, associated with kidney stones and mood disturbances, and surprisingly—osteoporosis.

Coenzyme Q_{10}

This naturally occurring nutrient is a powerful antioxidant, boosting the immune system, as well as guarding cells against aging and oxidative damage from highly unstable molecules called free radicals. It's important to test for coenzyme Q_{10} (CoQ_{10}) deficiency in the blood, particularly in patients with degenerative conditions such as congestive heart failure, chronic fatigue, kidney failure, and Parkinson's disease.

Essential Fatty Acid Profile*

Research now suggests that the single most important test for ascertaining an individual's risk for sudden cardiac death is an essential fatty acid (EFA) blood test that reveals the level of omega-3 oils in red blood cells.[8,9] EFAs or "good fats" are necessary for proper functioning of the cardiovascular, immune, nervous, and reproductive systems and cannot be manufactured by the body. Rather, they must be obtained via supplements and proper diet. Inadequate essential fatty acid levels correlate with schizophrenia, bipolar disease, and depression. In addition, low omega-3 intake may play a role in inflammatory diseases like arthritis, lupus, emphysema, and multiple sclerosis.

Antioxidant Levels

Some labs now offer new, advanced tests to evaluate an individual's antioxidant status. One popular test measures the level of cell-damaging lipid peroxides produced by free radicals. Since antioxidants, like vitamins C and E, shield the body from free radicals, getting a handle on your status can help you improve your diet and supplement program.

Hormonal Balance

As we age, subtle shifts in the production of various hormones can result in everything from depression to autoimmune diseases. These tests allow you to accurately detect hormone imbalances and right them with natural hormone therapies:

DHEA*

Dehydroepiandrosterone, or DHEA, is a natural hormone produced by the adrenal glands that declines with age. The DHEA blood test is particularly recommended for patients who may be DHEA-deficient, including those suffering from fatigue, autoimmune conditions, depression, chronic stress, low sex drive, adrenal "burnout," and those who have taken steroid medications. It's also a good measure of biological aging. If a deficiency is uncovered, taking DHEA supplements can improve mood and energy and even ameliorate autoimmune diseases, like lupus.

Testosterone and "Free" Testosterone Tests

Both men and women require testosterone, in differing amounts, for optimal health, energy, mood, sexual performance, and physical appearance. While the traditional testosterone blood test measures total testosterone levels in the body and can reveal severe deficiencies, only a measurement of "free" testosterone (the portion not bound to proteins that's hormonally active) can uncover more subtle imbalances.

Estrogen and Progesterone Tests

Adequate levels of these key female hormones are essential to a woman's well-being and can be determined through a blood test. This is particularly important for women over thirty-five, many of whom suffer from excessive estrogen and inadequate progesterone. This imbalance can lead to emotional volatility and anxiety, unstable blood sugar and carb cravings, weight gain (especially around the hips), rosacea, headaches, PMS, infertility, and heavy or irregular menstruation.

Cortisol (Adrenal Stress Index)

Levels of the stress hormone cortisol, manufactured by the adrenal glands, vary according to a set pattern throughout the day (levels are highest in the morning and gradually taper off at night). Common blood tests offered by endocrinologists are good at detecting serious diseases where production of cortisol soars or plummets, such as hypoglycemia. But subtle abnormalities reflecting chronic low-grade stress are harder to detect. The Adrenal Stress Index assesses minute abnormalities in adrenal function throughout the day by measuring cortisol levels every four hours until evening.

Allergy and Food Intolerance

The following tests are extremely accurate in uncovering allergies and intolerances to food and other environmental substances that can lie behind an array of serious health problems:

IgE RAST (Radio-Allergosorbent Test) Inhalants

This blood test provides a quick method for assessing the presence and extent of allergies to dust, mold, trees, grass, and weeds—environmental irritants that, when inhaled, trigger nasal congestion, chronic sinusitis, asthma, fatigue, headaches, and "brain-fog."

Skin Testing for Foods, Inhalants, and Candida

Positive results on the IgE RAST test (above) usually require further skin testing. Once allergies are confirmed, I like to treat them using sublingual drops, tiny extracts of symptom-triggering foods, inhalants, and candida (a yeast-like fungus in the gastrointestinal tract that can overgrow). Patients have achieved relief from such diverse conditions as respiratory problems, gastrointestinal disturbances, fatigue, fibromyalgia (generalized pain), headaches, arthritis, and skin maladies.

IgG RAST Test

This blood test identifies food intolerances responsible for a wide array of health problems. Among them: fatigue, joint and muscle pain, headaches, inflammatory problems, skin disorders, urinary and gastrointestinal symptoms (including irritable bowel syndrome), and even behavioral problems. The IgG RAST test focuses not on immediate reactions like classic nut or shellfish allergies, which can lead to anaphylaxis (a life-threatening allergic reaction), but rather on more insidious slow reactions that cumulatively challenge immune system function and can be alleviated by eliminating culprit foods.

Anti-Gliadin Antibody Test

This blood test detects sensitivity to gluten (wheat, rye, barley, and certain other grains), which can result in celiac sprue, a chronic disease that interferes with the absorption of nutrients in food. While true celiac sprue can only be conclusively diagnosed with an intestinal biopsy, the anti-gliadin antibody test often offers clues about whether a trial gluten-free diet is warranted.

Even gluten-intolerant patients who aren't suffering from overt symptoms of celiac sprue can experience abdominal bloating or pain, diarrhea, constipation, gaseousness, and acid reflux. Other symptoms include chronic sinusitis, asthma, skin disorders, fatigue, joint pains, mouth ulcers, bone pain, osteoporosis, iron deficiency anemia, abnormal menses in women, and infertility. And because gluten triggers immune system problems, any autoimmune disease, including those affecting the nervous system like multiple sclerosis or peripheral neuropathy (numbness and tingling of extremities), can also be related to gluten intolerance. In susceptible individuals, gluten may even set the stage for certain cancers.[10]

Brain and Nervous System

The following test helps uncover neurotransmitter imbalances that sometimes lead to less than optimal brain and nervous system functioning:

Neurotransmitter Profile

Neurotransmitters are chemicals produced by neurons to transmit signals throughout the nervous system. Imbalances of any neurotransmitter, including serotonin, epinephrine, norepinephrine (adrenalin), dopamine, and GABA can trigger depression, anxiety, fatigue, ADD, insomnia, migraines, and fibromyalgia. By analyzing morning urine, a nutritionally oriented doctor can recommend specific nutrient support to right these imbalances.

Bone Health

Get an early start on preventing age-related bone loss with these tests:

DEXA Scan

Dual energy x-ray absorptiometry is the main test used to screen for osteoporosis. The DEXA test yields a T-score, a positive or a negative number that indicates whether bone density is higher or lower than that of the average twenty-five-year-old woman (a T-score of less than −2.5 means osteoporosis).

The DEXA scan is recommended for women over the age of sixty-five, or for those at special risk (such as individuals who've used steroids or gone through early menopause without hormone replacement). However, I encourage women to take the test earlier, around fifty, so that corrective measures can be taken before bone loss has progressed too far. I also recommend the test for men over seventy, or where special risk factors suggest premature weakening of bone.

NTx Test

Obsessively rechecking your DEXA every few months for bone density changes is a little like watching the hour hand on your watch—nothing much changes if you look too often. A test called the urine N-telopeptide cross-links (NTx) is relatively inexpensive and can give an interim clue about the *rate* at which bone is being degraded. The test measures the level of proteins that leach from the bones when osteoporosis is accelerated and can also be used to gauge the effectiveness of measures undertaken to slow osteroporosis, like medications, nutritional support, and exercise.

In the next chapter, we'll build on the steps laid out here for maintaining optimal health by getting a full physical workup and explore ways to ensure the best care if you do become ill.

What to Do When You're Chronically Ill

Consider these facts about chronic disease:

• Each year approximately seven out of ten deaths in the United States (1.7 million) are caused by chronic conditions, such as cardiovascular disease, cancer, and diabetes.

• The prolonged course of illness from these conditions results in extended pain and suffering, limited mobility, and decreased quality of life for about 90 million Americans.

• Chronic diseases account for more than 75 percent of U.S. medical expenditures.

• More than 60 percent of people over sixty-five suffer from some form of cardiovascular disease. Half of all men and two-thirds of all women older than seventy have arthritis. By 2030, 70 million Americans (one in five) will be over sixty-five—meaning more people than ever living with chronic ailments.

• People who are overweight or obese are also more vulnerable to chronic conditions, including heart disease, diabetes, high blood pressure, arthritis-related disabilities, and some cancers. From 1987 to 2000, overweight and obesity increased dramatically—nearly 59 million adults are now obese, and the percentage of young people who are overweight has more than doubled in the last twenty years. Keep in mind, these are "real" increases in weight and not simply the result of number shifting due to the National Heart Lung and Blood Institute's revised obesity guidelines described in Chapter 4.

- The annual cost of obesity-related diseases in the United States is about $117 billion.

Certainly these statistics are alarming. Chronic diseases are among the most prevalent and costly health problems in this country. But they are also among the most *preventable*. In fact, adopting healthy behaviors, such as eating nutritious foods, being physically active, and avoiding tobacco use, can fend off or control the devastating effects of most "lifestyle" diseases. And not just in younger people. While the risk for disease and disability rises with age, poor health is not an inevitable consequence of growing older. Indeed, people with a healthy lifestyle have half the risk for disability that those with poorer health habits have.

I say all this for two reasons: One, as noted, the best barrier against chronic disease is—and always has been—prevention. Far fewer people would need the advice in this book if they just ate well, exercised, and didn't smoke. However, most of us, if we live long enough, will eventually face some sort of chronic health problem.

The good news is that conventional medicine has come a long way in acknowledging the role of "lifestyle" factors in chronic disease and is now taking a page from alternative medicine's prevention playbook. Even the federal government has gotten into the act with its National Center for Chronic Disease Prevention and Health Promotion, a division of the Centers for Disease Control (CDC). Even so, mainstream medicine—with its chief emphasis on high-tech interventions and drug therapies—still has a ways to go. Holistic and alternative medicine, on the other hand, has long placed chronic disease prevention and reversal at the top of its priority list, and is well situated with resources already in place to help America accomplish its critical health agenda.

Which brings me to my second point: Chronic disease is no longer an "either/or" proposition, requiring patients to choose either a conventional approach or an alternative approach. Both contribute important healing components. Mainstream medicine's potent new high-tech therapies have increasingly turned many health problems that were once killers, like cancer, into chronic conditions. But these treatments can also carry powerful side effects.

Enhancing the impact of conventional therapies and mitigating their effects via diet and other holistic treatments—a true integrative approach—is now more crucial than ever. Indeed, this is the main reason why I wrote this book. It's also the central theme of this chapter, which will explore the key role chronically ill patients can play in helping their physicians sort through various CAM and conventional options to decide the best course of treatment.

THE NEW CHRONIC CARE

The notion that two medical approaches are better than one was driven home to me early in my career. When I started my medical training a mere twenty-five years ago, many diseases (the vast majority of which were chronic in my chosen field of internal medicine) lay well beyond the reach of a conventional medicine fix.

During my residency, I often thought of myself as an emergency worker—a fireman sliding down the pole and extinguishing blazes. The analogy was an apt reflection of my surroundings at that time: New York City's Bronx borough was rapidly sliding downhill, a casualty of poverty-born arson. I could look out the hospital window almost daily and view impressive columns of smoke rising from drab, deserted neighborhoods—an ongoing visual reminder of the medicine I was being taught to practice. Yes, there was the drama of lifesaving interventions, but also frustration and monotony in caring for the chronic disorders of "recidivist" patients.

Today, much has changed. New "targeted" treatment technologies and drugs, such as monoclonal antibodies, exist for chronic conditions, like severe rheumatoid arthritis, psoriasis, colitis, multiple sclerosis, and lupus. Special "assist pumps" can now be surgically installed to bolster failing hearts. Even obesity is increasingly treated via bariatric weight-loss surgery that seals off the stomach to reduce how much is eaten.

The trouble is, though, not only are the costs of these treatments enormous, but they can also result in severe and lasting side effects. Even advocates of high-tech medicine recognize their limitations, as this recent quote from a *New England Journal of Medicine* article on bariatric surgery suggests:

> The increasing prevalence of obesity not only in adults but also in children and adolescents—indeed, bariatric surgery is now being considered a potential pediatric intervention—indicate the urgent need to implement effective preventive interventions, beginning early in life, to improve dietary habits and increase physical activity. Bariatric surgery is currently the most successful approach to "rescuing" patients with severe obesity and reversing or preventing the development of several diseases associated with obesity. It would be an even greater success to make these procedures unnecessary.[1]

Feeling Lousy

The truth is, many chronic diseases—particularly those vague, hard-to-diagnose complaints that many patients report (often early warning signs of more serious diseases in the making)—still sit well beyond the reach of conventional medicine. Indeed, for all its dazzle and progress, mainstream medicine has yet to rescue many of us from chronic unhealthiness—and probably never will by itself.

Consider a recent study from the CDC suggesting that the health-related quality of life of most Americans (including their physical and mental health, plus their ability to do their usual activities) has deteriorated over the past few years.[2] On average, those surveyed reported that their physically unhealthy days per month increased from 3.0 in 1993 to 3.5 days in 2001, their mentally unhealthy days rose from 2.9 to 3.4 days, and limited-activity days increased from 1.6 to 2.0 days. The percentage of U.S. adults rating their health as fair or poor also rose from 13.4 percent in 1993 to 15.5 percent in 2001. This is progress?

Should people just resign themselves to feeling lousy? Are the unprecedented wellness expectations of aging baby boomers unrealistic? Certainly, I see my share of patients suffering from chronic "unwellness." Not yet diagnosed with specific, treatable maladies, they are the walking wounded, in limbo between suboptimal health and definable disease. Sometimes I tell these patients, with some irony: "You're auditioning for a disease, but fortunately you haven't quite landed the part yet."

Many of them have been cajoled by their doctors to lower their expectations. "I feel your pain," they're told. "My back/stomach/knees hurt, too. But that's how it is when you're forty-four (or fifty-six, or sixty-three, or eighty)." It's not that doctors want to discourage patients from seeking peak wellness, it's just that many don't know what more can be achieved. They aren't operating with a full stockpile of remedies—the tools of a true CAM approach.

Patient Tenacity

The plight of one such patient illustrates the potential benefits that CAM can bring to chronic, poorly defined ill health.

Aurora was forty-eight when she came to see me and felt many years older than her chronological age. She complained of being "tired all the time"—the title of one my books. To her credit, she maintained a great mental attitude in the face of adversity. Despite repeated unsuccessful attempts by mainstream doctors to find the cause of her problems, she still retained faith in her ability to unravel the cause of her fatigue and other troubling symptoms. In fact, her training as a registered dietician finally prompted her to seek my services after years of floundering.

Her difficulties had begun when she gave birth prematurely to her last child. Her weight soared seventy pounds during the pregnancy, and afterward she was not able to take if off. Nor did her energy return to normal. Thyroid medication seemed to help, but her doctors withdrew it—despite her weight gain, lethargy, dry skin, and puffy features—because her thyroid blood tests were only borderline low.

Over the years, she developed allergies, nasal congestion, and itchy skin. Her stomach began to hurt chronically, and she was found to be anemic. Acid blockers didn't help, and she took iron pills to no avail. As she approached menopause, she began to feel even worse. Her primary care doctor couldn't help, but urged her to take a statin drug to lower her elevated cholesterol.

When I saw Aurora, I suspected I could make her better by employing my usual bag of tricks—strict adherence to the Salad and Salmon Diet to control her looming Syndrome X; natural thyroid to accelerate her sluggish metabolism; identification and treatment of food intolerances which might trigger her allergy and gastrointestinal symptoms; and appropriate nutritional supplements to reignite her flagging energy. But I wasn't entirely prepared for what I found. (See Chapter 6 for details on my Salad and Salmon Diet.)

Aurora turned out to have celiac disease, a classic nutritional condition, involving gluten intolerance, that's often missed in conventional workups. The average patient diagnosed with celiac disease is misdiagnosed for at least a decade, sometimes two or three. What makes celiac hard to diagnose is that its symptoms are subtle and numerous: fatigue, chronic malnutrition (including iron deficiency), fertility problems and miscarriages (Aurora had miscarried prior to delivery of her last child), autoimmune maladies, and gastrointestinal symptoms. In obvious cases of celiac, the patient suffers from chronic diarrhea and becomes emaciated. But researchers are coming to recognize that a fairly high percentage of patients with celiac actually defy the stereotype. They may be overweight, like Aurora, even constipated.

We embarked on a treatment plan specifically tailored to her particular health needs. I placed Aurora on a strict gluten-free diet, supplemented her with nutrients she was depleted in, and began administering some natural thyroid. The results were remarkable. Aurora's energy surged, the pounds melted off as her metabolism was rekindled, and her stomach pain abated. Within six months, her nasal congestion and itchy skin were gone. She no longer took to her bed after returning home from work and cooking dinner for her family, and even began an exercise program. Her cholesterol dipped 80 points, and after years of anemia, her iron levels climbed to normal. Had it not been for Aurora's tenacity in pursuing the true causes of her malaise, and stepping outside the standard medical paradigm for extra help, she might have been relegated to the ranks of the chronically ill for the rest of her life.

DECIPHERING SYMPTOMS

Being over fifty is an art—a tricky balance between prudence and constructive denial about all those aches and changes that seem to crop up with age. Your very survival is at stake, and no one knows your body better than you. But you must decide which symptoms call for action and which can safely be ignored or self-treated.

Some people are too attuned to subtle changes in how they feel, others, not enough. Sometimes this breaks along sex lines (though certainly not always), with men in stoic denial about symptoms and women tempted to call their doctor at the first sign of any ache or sneeze. Actually, both extremes—chronic health worry and stubborn denial—place your health at risk.

The key to successful coping with any bodily discomfort is to properly assess it and place it in context. All symptoms (feelings) and signs (physical manifestations) lie along a spectrum of normal (not menacing) to abnormal (something to see your doctor about). The trick is to match each symptom and sign with its proper medical implication. Unfortunately, this isn't always easy. Sometimes alarming symptoms indicate relatively minor problems, while barely discernible symptoms turn out to have whopper health consequences. Here's an example I sometimes give patients:

Occasionally, someone will have terrible abdominal cramps, and unpredictable bowel movements, ranging from constipation to urgency. These signs are attention-riveting, to say the least, and warrant an immediate and thorough medical evaluation. However, often after a full GI (gastrointestinal) workup, including stool tests, blood tests, scoping, CT scans, MRIs, and now even swallowable mini-cameras, nothing is found. The patient is diagnosed with irritable bowel syndrome (IBS), told not to worry, and urged to pick up some Metamucil on the way home.

IBS is just one example of a condition with very bothersome symptoms that's ultimately not dangerous. I sometimes humorously reassure my patients: "Don't worry, you'll live a long and miserable life (that is, in the unlikely event that my regimen of diet modification, stress reduction, herbs, meditation, acupuncture, biofeedback, and probiotics fails to improve your condition!)"

On the other hand, picture this scenario: A patient sits down to a painless, normal bowel movement, and notices bright red blood in the toilet. She is alarmed at first, but since she feels fine, she flushes the toilet and puts it out of her mind. Unfortunately, finding blood in your stool is often a red flag for colon cancer.

In the first situation, the event (symptoms or signs) looms large, but the connotation is ultimately insignificant. In the second scenario, the event seems trivial, but the *connotation* may be dire.

$$\text{EVENT} \longrightarrow \text{CONNOTATION}$$
$$\text{EVENT} \longrightarrow \textbf{CONNOTATION}$$

If the woman who sees red blood ignores her symptoms, the potential delay in diagnosing a growing colon cancer could mean the difference between early surgery to eliminate it or death from metastatic cancer found too late.

But there's an additional wrinkle. Potentially dire symptoms that shouldn't be ignored, like new-onset headaches, blood in the urine or stool, even chest pain, are often not associated with serious conditions. They just need to be checked out, particularly past age forty-five. A lot of these are sure to be near misses—alarming symptoms that don't ultimately translate into a calling card from the Grim Reaper. But without a balanced perspective on all these weird bodily aches and twinges, a person really can live a long and miserable life in constant dread.

Deciding What to Do

Faced with new symptoms, there are essentially three ways to go:

1. **See a doctor.**

2. **Watchful waiting.** Monitoring symptoms to see whether they abate or get worse over time. As a rule, benign conditions are self-limited, and dangerous problems recur and mount in intensity.

3. **Self-care.** Includes eating right, exercise, vitamin/mineral/herb supplements, and stress management. This approach is very much in line with the tenets of complementary and alternative medicine, which emphasizes patient empowerment.

Deciding which approach is best requires boosting your health literacy so you can "triage" health problems. Books like this and radio programs like mine can go a long way toward helping the public better sort out health issues, from minor to major (see Chapter 3 for more on medical literacy). The following websites also offer help in sifting through symptoms and deciding which require medical attention and which don't:

• **AllRefer.com Symptoms Guide:** http://health.allrefer.com/health/symptoms.html. Includes step-by-step instructions for evaluating symptoms, from blood in urine and heartburn to abdominal pain and skin rash.

• **MyElectronicMD.com:** www.myelectronicmd.com. Online self-screening tool allows you to click on body parts experiencing symptoms to learn about possible causes and what to do.

• **WebMD Symptom Checker:** http://my.webmd.com/medical_information/check_symptoms/default.htm?z=1727_00000_1110_dp_03). Similar online self-screening tool, allowing you to click on areas of the body experiencing problems.

As you decipher the meaning of symptoms, it's important to keep a few facts in mind. First, many diseases exist within a particular context. For example, if you're over fifty and have high cholesterol and blood pressure, it's not unreason-

able to conclude that chest pains might signal heart disease, requiring an immediate visit to your doctor. However, for twenty-somethings with a clean bill of
health, vague chest pressure is more likely to be innocuous indigestion, muscle
strain, or stress. Watchful waiting and a little self-care are probably a safe bet. That
said, though: don't automatically ignore symptoms, imagining that you're invul-
nerable. Even the youngest and healthiest among us sometimes get sick.

SPEAKING DOCTOR-ESE

If you end up going to a doctor, here are some communication tips to make your
time more productive. First, don't go in with high expectations for a rapid or dramatic resolution to the problem, particularly if symptoms are chronic and vague.
A series of visits might be required, and a realistic preliminary goal could involve
little more than establishing an orderly process of testing (or even waiting). I
notice that engineers, computer types, and mechanics have the biggest problem
with the messy imprecision of medicine. I say if it took hours on the phone with
Indian-accented technicians in Bangalore to exorcise my computer demons after
a recent spyware attack, imagine how long it might take to clear up an enigmat-
ic health issue?

Also, when presenting your problem to the doctor (who typically has only a
few minutes to see you), aim for brevity and saliency. A 1999 study found that
patients are typically interrupted by their doctors twenty-three seconds into
explaining their problems.[3] In fact, few patients actually get to finish describing
their concerns, resulting in missed data that could lead to a better diagnosis.

To improve your doctor's chances of getting all your vital information, resist
the temptation to tell your story chronologically from the very beginning ("I had
my tonsils out in the sixth grade . . ."). Some patients seem to want to withhold
the plot twists and the surprise ending, as if they were savoring a whodunit or
describing a movie.

Instead spill the beans and tell everything up front ("I've experienced three
weeks of worsening stomach burning" or "five days of pain when I take a deep
breath" or "I've been diagnosed with lupus"). Try to convey what your symptoms
feel like rather than offering a diagnosis. For example, saying, "I have cramping
pain under my right ribcage which comes and goes, and it's frequently worse after
fatty meals," is more valuable than saying "My gallbladder hurts." Once you've
provided the main plotline, you can fill your doctor in on specific details he or
she may find relevant ("It all started when I broke up with my boyfriend" or "I've
been unusually thirsty"). See "Explaining Your Symptoms" on page 86 for more
communication tips.

That said, though, remember that you may not need to recount every seemingly salient detail, especially during the first visit. Even doctors can be over-

whelmed by too much information. Keep in mind the old adage, "less is more." I notice with each passing year in practice that my capabilities in "pattern recognition" are constantly improving.

This idea has been proven in studies on perception: when researchers try to experimentally blind certain parts of the eye with special vision-limiting goggles, the brain's pattern-recognition software overrides it, allowing people to identify familiar objects—even with only minimal ability to see. So don't despair if your doctor doesn't take in everything with one fell swoop. Give most of us a few choice pieces of information and our minds are likely to automatically apply a familiar template, based on extensive experience, to fill in the gaps and hopefully clinch a diagnosis.

Finally, don't be afraid to offer your own personal opinion about what might be causing your problem. Some physicians find this annoying or threatening, but the fact remains that with certain poorly recognized conditions, like Lyme disease, parasitic infections, or celiac disease, studies reveal it is often patients who first alert doctors to these possibilities. While your physician may not concur with your opinion, the very least you should expect is respectful listening and a reasoned explanation about why it isn't plausible. See "Practice Tips for Doctors" on page 90 for ways doctors can use "narrative medicine" techniques to better process what patients are saying.

What to Bring

In addition to describing your symptoms, you might also organize your records, and if possible, supply a simple chronology of your disease in outline form. Many of my wonkier patients are adept at creating spreadsheets, and I appreciate their efforts to present me with a quick visual aid. But keep it simple. Your goal is to inform, not overwhelm your doctor.

Be sure to provide the names and addresses of other doctors you've been seeing. This will make it easier to stay in contact with them and to order medical records. *Always* keep comprehensive medical records in a file at home—it is your right to obtain copies of all tests you've undergone, and copies of consultation notes in which doctors summarize their opinions. In most states, it's even your right to obtain handwritten notes, although decoding scribbled doctor-ese often proves formidable.

If you're seeing a new physician or seeking a second opinion, don't assume you shouldn't bring your medical records. Many patients mistakenly believe a new doctor will be confused or unfairly influenced by prior consultation notes and test results, and won't be able to offer a fresh, unbiased perspective. However, seeing patients outside the context of their prior care not only provides an incomplete picture, but it can also draw out the process of identifying what's wrong while

EXPLAINING YOUR SYMPTOMS

Martin Tracy, a sixty-nine-year-old retired accountant, suffered on and off for months from severe fatigue, arthritis-like joint pain, headaches, and mood swings. At first he assumed he was suffering from repeated bouts of the flu. But as the symptoms multiplied and worsened, he decided to do some research. His self-diagnosis—based on careful detective work and a "gut" feeling—surprised even his wife. Martin was convinced he had Lyme disease. His doctor wasn't so sure:

Martin: Doc, the symptoms come and go—weeks without anything, then they are back—headaches, sore joints, achiness, fatigue. Lately, the pain seems to move around my body, and it's getting worse. I've lost my appetite, I'm forgetful, and can hardly get out of bed some days. This probably sounds crazy, but I think I might have Lyme disease.

Dr. Beltzner: Marty, these symptoms could indicate any number of conditions. Besides, you never found a tick or a bull's-eye rash, did you?

Martin: Well, not exactly, but take a look at this symptom timeline I put together. I was gardening a lot last summer. Around July 4, I noticed large circular blotches on my arms and legs. I assumed it was poison ivy or a heat rash. I also got a low-grade fever about that time. I never found a tick, and the rash and fever disappeared after a few days, but in retrospect I'm convinced it was the beginning of Lyme disease.

Dr. Beltzner: Perhaps . . . but the Lyme rash is usually a single red ring at the site of the tick bite.

Martin: According to my research, Doc, not every rash is alike and some people don't even get one.

Dr. Beltzner: Marty, let's test you for something more likely, like rheumatoid arthritis, before we start worrying about Lyme disease.

Martin: Doc, I feel pretty certain about this—call it a hunch. If it's Lyme disease, I'd like to get started on treatment right away.

Dr. Beltzner finally agreed and was surprised when the test came back positive. Through antibiotics and a regimen of supplements and exercise, Martin's symptoms gradually disappeared and he returned to full health.

new tests are performed (sometimes redundantly) and records are ordered. We'll discuss second opinions in more detail later in this chapter.

Remember, too, that when visiting a new doctor for the first time, it's okay to gently probe for his or her views on your use of complementary and alternative methods. This "vetting" process needn't be exhaustive at this time, particularly if you're seeking a specialist to do a delicate operation or administer a high-tech conventional therapy. But if you're looking for a long-term care advocate and partner to unravel your complex medical challenges, it's best to root out any hostility against CAM from the get-go. Ask directly if your doctor is willing to help you objectively evaluate the pros and cons of alternative approaches you wish to explore. Rage, sarcasm, and impatience are all inappropriate reactions.

Decision to Test

If your doctor suggests additional tests to help make a diagnosis, recognize that you—the patient—remain the ultimate arbiter of what happens to your body. Recall from the previous chapter that a decision to test is often a decision to treat. For example, if you experience some shortness of breath after mild physical exertion and your doctor recommends an angiogram, this could lead to insertion of a stent to prop open your artery or coronary bypass surgery if any blockage is found. Your doctor might even use charged language ("You have an obstructed blood vessel—we call that a 'widow-maker'!").

Of course, the test or ensuing treatments might well be necessary. But your doctor may omit crucial information that could lead you to choose differently. For instance, in Canada and England where stringent cost-containment measures often deny patients easy, immediate access to angiograms, heart disease death rates are comparable to those in the United States. In other words, getting an angiogram doesn't necessarily boost your odds against dying from heart disease.

What's more, your doctor may also neglect to tell you about alternatives, such as chelation therapy or Dr. Dean Ornish's successful program to reverse coronary artery blockage with diet and lifestyle changes (see Chapter 6).

Therefore, when scheduled for a round of tests, be sure to ask these key questions:

- What exactly is this test designed to find out?
- How will the results ultimately affect the management of my problem?

If you're suffering, for instance, from mild stomach pain, your doctor might order an upper endoscopy, which requires you to swallow a thin, lighted tube for picture taking inside your esophagus, stomach, and duodenum. If this fairly invasive test is only likely to confirm a minor problem that both you and your doctor already suspect, it may not be necessary. Likewise, if your doctor is only going to prescribe acid blockers regardless of your test results, you might skip it, as well. (Note: Cases of persistent or severe pain *do* demand additional evaluation.)

Instead, you could suggest postponing the test, and instead trying a healthy diet for a while, along with medication. If your pain responds, you might just defer the test altogether.

If You Don't Understand . . . Ask

Medicine has a rarified language of its own that can intimidate even the most medically literate patient. As we saw in Chapter 3, doctors often attempt to arrive at a diagnosis via a process of elimination, often ruling out the most unlikely—and frightening—possibilities first using highly technical and unfamiliar "medicalese." For patients that can mean a slew of very scary sounding test results and medical terms that may not actually be as dire as they first seem—such as "refractory" (hard to treat), "nonspecific" (no obvious disease causing the symptoms), "contraindicated" (not advised), "spontaneous involution" (disappearance of symptoms on their own) and "dysgeusia" (loss of taste or taste abnormality).

If you don't understand something your doctor says, ask him or her to rephrase it in plain English. It's not that your doctor is deliberately trying to frighten or confuse you; it's just that "med-speak" is probably second nature. Repeat back your understanding of what was said to clear up any lingering confusion or misinterpretation. This will help you get a better handle on your medical condition and ensure that you follow your treatment plan properly. Buy a good medical dictionary to help you decipher medical jargon and take more control of your care. See Resources for Patients for online medical dictionaries.

DON'T BE THE FIRST ON YOUR BLOCK . . .

Once you're diagnosed, devising a treatment plan is the next order of business—a complex and emotionally charged task for many patients. Do you go the low-tech or high-tech route? Drugs or herbal remedies? Surgery or lifestyle interventions? Or some combination of both?

Whatever you and your doctor decide, just remember that there's a lot of hype out there, requiring a methodical, reasonable approach to sort the "too-good-to-be-true" from the "likely-to-succeed."

This is particularly so for patients with challenging medical conditions who are often irresistibly drawn to the dramatic claims of new drugs and experimental treatments. But the recent ballyhooed withdrawal of several "breakthrough" drugs and the collapse of clinical trials involving radical new surgical techniques should provide a lesson to eager patients—unless a therapy represents a last-ditch attempt at survival, it's best to wait on the sidelines awhile until it has a more established track record of effectiveness and safety.

Years ago, I read an interesting article by health journalist Gary Schwitzer, in which he cited seven "loaded" words reporters shouldn't use in covering medical news—a takeoff on comedian George Carlin's list of seven words you're not allowed to say over the airwaves.

When sorting through treatment options, be wary of any described with one of Schwitzer's "taboo" terms: *cure, miracle, breakthrough, promising, dramatic, hope,* and *victim.* All are ill-defined and vague and can mean different things to different people. For instance, does every "breakthrough" pan out as a "miracle" cure? Or do some "promising" treatments ultimately fail to meet expectations because of side effects or lack of effectiveness?

To determine whether an experimental drug or treatment is a flash-in-the-pan or a legitimate possibility, visit the CenterWatch Clinical Trials Listing Service (www.centerwatch.com) or ClinicalTrials.gov (http://clinicaltrials.gov) for thousands of active government and industry-sponsored clinical trials and names of drugs under investigation.

Not Rocket Science

If you feel bewildered by your medical options, try a tried-and-true concept that doctors resort to all the time—the risk/benefit equation. Some patients by their nature are risk averse. Others are enthusiasts, oblivious to danger. Find out where you reside on the continuum, and compile a comprehensive list of upside benefits and downside risks for every therapy you're contemplating. Do your research, talk to your doctor, take time to make a reasoned decision—then act. In some cases, you may find that you want to try a gentler option first, like those listed below, before opting for a stronger, more expensive conventional therapy that's potentially hazardous and hasn't been definitively proven effective:

- Glucosamine versus Vioxx in osteoarthritis;

- Fish oil versus lung reduction surgery in Chronic Obstructive Pulmonary Disease (COPD);

- Curcumin and vitamin E versus Aricept in Alzheimer's disease.

With the first two examples above, Vioxx and lung reduction surgery were abandoned after rigorous trials showed their risks outweighed modest benefits. In the latter example, new trials are showing that Aricept is at best marginally effective in delaying the progression of Alzheimer's disease.

Keep in mind that medicine isn't rocket science, and that few decisions can be made unequivocally. While this is scary for many patients who want certainty, the fact that medicine can be imprecise may make the decision-making process less fraught with second-guessing and doubt. I tell patients that the closer the call,

PRACTICE TIPS FOR DOCTORS: NARRATIVE MEDICINE

If your doctor knows only medicine,
you can be sure he knows not even medicine.

—MARK TWAIN

Puzzled by the complex stories patients often told about their symptoms, Dr. Rita Charon began taking English courses to learn more about how stories are structured, narrated, and understood. Not long afterward, she had the following revelation:

> I realized that the narrative skills I was learning in my English studies made me a better doctor. I could listen to what my patients tell me with a greater ability to follow the narrative thread of their story, to recognize the governing images and metaphors, to adopt the patients' or family members' points of view, to identify the sub-texts present in all stories, to interpret one story in the light of others told by the same teller. Moreover, the better I was as "reader" of what my patients told me, the more deeply moved I myself was by their predicament, making more of my self available to patients as I tried to help.[4]

The result was a new branch of medical communication, called narrative medicine. (Dr. Charon is now director of the narrative medicine program at the College of Physicians and Surgeons of Columbia University). The aim is to help doctors understand what patients' symptoms represent for them and collaborate on a healing path that makes sense for the patient.

A strange incident occurred during my own medical training, which brought home the importance of listening to patient narratives. A young woman was admitted to our floor with a bewildering array of symptoms and inexplicable blood-test abnormalities. She was in pain and distraught. Dozens of specialists paraded in and out of her room, but she continued to deteriorate.

the more likely it's a matter of a coin toss: six of one, a half dozen of another. In other words, few treatments offer a 100 percent guarantee.

As you decide, pay attention to your instincts. As popular author and patient-empowerment guru Dr. Bernie Siegel notes in his writings, patients need to believe in their doctors and their prescribed course of treatment. Passive patients who simply abdicate all decision making to their doctors or loved ones do worse

Finally, I naively inquired what she thought was wrong. She was of Caribbean background and believed in the Santeria religion. Somehow she communicated to me in Spanish that she believed her malevolent in-laws were trying to poison her. "I feel the poison in my stomach going into my veins," she confided.

Her medical team's immediate response was to give her a psychiatric evaluation and administer antipsychotic medications. But to no avail. However, the notion that she felt poisoned stuck with me. There are a group of rare hereditary diseases, called porphyrias, which can be triggered by various drugs, dietary changes, or even hormonal fluctuations. Patients often experience perplexing symptoms, such as pain and psychiatric aberrations. What's most interesting, though, is that these diseases spring from the accumulation of toxic metabolites, called porphyrins, in people who lack the enzymes to break them down—causing them to feel like they're being poisoned. After discussing the possibility at rounds, we called a specialist, performed some tests, and confirmed the diagnosis.

Here are some narrative medicine strategies that can help doctors gain more insight into their patients:

- **Ask patients what they think is going on.** And then take a few moments to really listen—even if what they say initially strikes you as medically implausible. At best, patients will provide clues to the origin of their disease; at worst, even if patients assign their maladies to a prior alien abduction (even I draw the line somewhere!), you'll gain some insight into their belief system about healing and be able to collaborate more effectively on a treatment plan.

- **Encourage patients to provide a personal perspective.** For example, I often ask patients to fill me in on their lives. If they're artists, I ask to see a portfolio of their work. If they're grandparents, I want to know what role they play in caring for their grandkids. It's important to find out what patients are living for. This is different from glad-handing or hob-nobbing with your patients, which is ethically questionable, and usually results in weakening, rather than fortifying, the doctor-patient bond.

than quarrelsome, empowered patients who "bug" their physicians with questions. Doctors may have their backs to the wall because of time constraints in contemporary medicine, but in my opinion they should welcome patients who query them about multiple treatment options because patients who feel heard ultimately fare better no matter what therapy they end up choosing.

The good news is that hundreds of drug-supplement reactions have now

been studied and well documented, and as often as not, many are actually beneficial. See Resources for Physicians and Resources for Patients for tools to check
possible interactions.

In subsequent chapters, we'll explore important drug-nutrient reactions per-
taining to specific conditions so you and your doctor can devise a safer, more
effective complementary healing plan.

GETTING A SECOND OPINION

There are times when a second—and even third opinion—is valuable (and imper-
ative), including when you don't agree with your doctor's diagnosis or treatment

---

UNCOVERING DRUG-SUPPLEMENT INTERACTIONS

Even if your physician is skeptical about your forays into natural medicine and
complementary self-care, there's one sure way to get his or her attention—mention the possibility of drug-supplement interactions. With growing acceptance of
natural products, new concerns are rising about possible unpredictable interactions between conventional drugs and supplements, including vitamins, minerals,
amino acids, and herbs. An estimated 15 million Americans are at risk for supple-
ment-drug interactions, particularly those with chronic conditions who take multiple medications.[5]

Reactions generally fall into three categories:

- **1+1 = 2 (Amplification):** When a supplement enhances the effectiveness of
a drug, either beneficially or harmfully. Well-known examples include the
effects of the now-banned herbal supplement ephedra and certain deconges-
tants or asthma medications, which taken together can cause dangerous spikes
in blood pressure, palpitations, insomnia, or anxiety.

- **1+1 = 0 (Interference):** When a supplement cancels out a drug's effects.
The antidepressant herb St. John's wort, for example, can counteract several medications, including immunosuppressant drugs designed to prevent organ rejec-
tion in transplant patients, certain AIDS drugs, and even oral contraceptives.

- **1+1 = (Wildcard!):** When combining a supplement and drug produces an
undesirable and unpredictable reaction (neither amplification nor cancellation)
via an indirect effect. An example is the combination of licorice (which can
cause the kidneys to excrete potassium) with the heart drug digoxin (which can
provoke dangerous heart arrhythmias when potassium levels are low).

recommendation or when a health problem recurs and you're seeking a new therapy that your physician isn't completely sold on. Granted, all doctors receive similar training, but each one is an individual with his or her own views on which treatments to recommend and how aggressive to be.

Unfortunately, getting a second opinion can be hard going for even the most intrepid patient.[6] Because your medical records might be scattered between medical offices and labs, you may have to visit each one individually to gather all the information needed. Hospitals and physicians are also increasingly reluctant to provide time-consuming second opinions, which net them little reimbursement.

The key is persistence. Call a local teaching hospital or medical society for names of physicians. You can also contact services, like Second Opinion Medical Information (www.physicians-background.com), which, for a fee, will conduct a background check on doctors you're considering, provide a list of other possible diagnoses, and locate the best hospital for your treatment.

One word of caution: While I welcome the new candor about doctors' and hospitals' track records, this information can be misinterpreted. For example, neurosurgeons who perform high-risk procedures are routinely sued—the price they pay for undertaking medically risky surgeries. So a neurosurgeon's malpractice record may not be a good benchmark of whether she or he is a competent doctor. Additionally, checking the death rate for say, heart surgery, at a particular hospital may be misleading: top-tier health facilities are often referral sources for higher-risk patients that smaller community hospitals aren't willing to take. For more on when and how to get a second opinion, turn to Resources for Patients. See Chapter 11 for tips on seeking a surgical second opinion.

A THIRD OPINION

That said, it's important, too, to remember that incisive, critical opinions and innovative approaches *can* also be offered by physicians outside a particular medical "guild." For a truly alternative perspective, some patients seek a third opinion from a complementary physician—many of whom are eclectics who may or may not be prestigiously boarded or have other advanced credentialing—but who are nevertheless highly qualified to offer significant care and treatment strategies. Some patients even decide to stay on permanently to pursue a CAM approach to their care. This concept is explored in more detail in John M. Fink's book *Third Opinion,* which lists the names, addresses, and phone numbers of alternative and complementary clinics around the world, plus the diseases they treat and therapies they use.

In addition, check out the American Holistic Health Association's Resource and Referral List at http://ahha.org/ahre.htm for professional organizations that provide referrals to qualified, licensed CAM practitioners. Here's a sampling:

- **American College for Advancement in Medicine.** 23121 Verdugo Dr., Suite 204, Laguna Hills, CA 92653; (888) 439-6891: www.acam.org. Free online and phone referrals to over 1,000 licensed holistic M.D. and D.O. members.

- **American Board of Holistic Medicine.** 1135 Makawao Ave., #230, Makawao, HI 96768; (808) 572-4616: www.holisticboard.org. Free referrals to over 650 M.D.s and D.O.s who are board-certified holistic physicians.

- **American Holistic Medical Association.** 12101 Menaul Blvd., NE, Suite C, Albuquerque, NM 87112; (505) 292-7788: www.holisticmedicine.org. Free online search or send $15 for directory of over 700 holistic M.D.s, D.O.s, and other holistic health providers with current unrestricted licenses.

AFTER TREATMENT

With chronic disease there's almost no such thing as a full or complete recovery. You may stop treatment, but you'll probably want to continue monitoring your condition for any signs of change, particularly a relapse or worsening of symptoms. Chances are you'll also want to adopt some secondary prevention strategies, such as taking supplements and exercising. (Secondary prevention means warding off recurrence of an existing condition. Primary prevention means avoiding it in the first place.)

This involves educating yourself about what to expect in the post-treatment phase (see "Uncovering Drug-Supplement Interactions" on page 92 for information on adverse reactions between certain drugs and dietary supplements) and maintaining an ongoing partnership with your doctor.

Talk to your physician about touching base periodically to update him or her on your condition. These "maintenance" checks can be done via a personal visit, phone, or email, and allow you to discuss changes in your health, as well as hammer out any needed adjustments to your medication or lifestyle strategies. Be sure to check with your doctor first about his or her preferred method of communicating and how often to get in touch.

The strategies outlined here and in Chapter 4 are designed to help you develop a proactive approach to disease prevention and health. We've discussed how to get a thorough physical, including a few non-conventional tests that can give you a heads up on potential health problems. We've also looked at ways to get the care you need when problems do arise and how to partner with your doctor on a healing plan. In the remaining chapters we'll help you tailor these strategies to specific health conditions.

Heart
Disease

Take another little piece of my heart now, baby!
Break another little bit of my heart now, darling . . .
—*PIECE OF MY HEART,* BY JANIS JOPLIN

In July 2004, ex-President Bill Clinton became the poster-boy for aggressive cardiac intervention. All the right ingredients were there: Clinton was demographically correct—no geezer by a long shot, he was the quintessential baby boomer. He was busy, powerful, and full of vitality, had access to all the right health information, good doctors, and primo health insurance. He talked a good "health" game, too—yet clung to a few favorite vices. A non-cigarette smoker, he wasn't averse to an occasional cigar. His efforts to eat right were almost as legendary as his hankerings for French fries. And exercise was more "show" than strict regimen (remember all those presidential photos of him gamely jogging through Washington). In other words, he was someone the 80 million boomers now coasting toward their prime cardiovascular risk years could easily identify with.

News of his impending cardiac crisis sent a dire message about the capriciousness of health. If this endearing embodiment of the boomer lifestyle could so unpredictably end up with heart disease, then *anyone* could.

The press played it like a "saved in the nick of time" story. "Clinton Likely Headed for Major Heart Attack," screamed the headlines. Even his doctor, Allan Schwartz, chief of cardiology at New York-Presbyterian Hospital/Columbia University Medical Center, declared triumphantly that only timely quadruple bypass surgery to re-route blood from his blocked arteries could save him.

Freshly outfitted with a clean set of coronaries, Clinton was pronounced "fixed"—headed down an open road with nothing but trouble-free mileage ahead. The script was made-to-order, and Clinton once again fulfilled his role as sentinel of his generation. In suburbs all across America, previously confident baby boomers paused to consider whether they, too, should check in with their cardiologists.

Sure, there were the usual calls for lifestyle change. Medical experts noted that

Clinton really should forgo those fries, as well as his cigars. And his exercise regimen needed to be more than a sporadic photo-op. But as with many celebrity
interventions (think David Letterman, Larry King), the whole thing still came off
like a paean to high-tech intervention. Not only did bypass surgery receive a
major plug, but so did cholesterol-lowering statin drugs (it turns out that Clinton
hadn't heeded his doctors' advice to take them).

As we all know now, there was a sequel to Clinton's "perfect" recovery story
line. A rare complication involving compression of his lung by fibrotic tissue
required a second operation. The ex-president recovered nicely, but the problems
he experienced exemplify a wide range of potential after-effects of heart surgery—everything from strokes and chronic thoracic pain, to post-surgical depression and cognitive impairment.

Even with this complication, though, I still fear that "success" stories like this
convince the public that all heart disease is a plumbing problem, that fate and
genes play bigger roles in determining who gets heart disease than personal
responsibility, and that salvation awaits in the cardiac-catheterization suite.

Indeed, this message permeates our culture. Widely aired TV ads for statin
drugs play to our fears that health is really out of our control. Recall the healthy-
looking, aging boomer types (blonde diva at a Hollywood premiere, muscular
gray fox by the poolside, and thin female surfer)—all presumably with high cholesterol—as they variously stumble, belly flop, and crash into surfboards to under-
score the arbitrariness of risk. The message: No one—no matter how attractive or
seemingly fit—is immune from heart problems.

In this chapter we'll attempt to cut through these misconceptions and medical hype and take an honest look at low-tech heart-disease prevention and treatment strategies that really work. We'll also explore current controversies and
potential interactions with conventional therapies that you'll want discuss with
your doctor.

FIVE LITTLE-KNOWN FACTS ABOUT HEART DISEASE

Research is beginning to show that many of our common conceptions about
heart disease are erroneous. The mechanical notion of heart disease as a "plumbing problem" is gradually being supplanted by more subtle notions of how the
disease originates and progresses. Here are some examples of how conventional
wisdom is changing.

  • **Fact one:** We spend enormous amounts, per capita, on our cardiac inter-
    ventions in America and get less bang for our buck than other Western nations.
    In fact, our health care spending for cardiovascular disease is the most lavish in
    the world, but our death rates have changed little over time. Indeed, recent

gains in our fight against heart disease are largely the result of more people giving up cigarettes, not wider availability of high-tech procedures. Granted, many of these interventions are good at alleviating certain symptoms, such as the chest discomfort and pain of angina, but they don't necessarily improve outcomes.

• **Fact two:** Statin drugs are both too-little and too-much used. That is, our current "paint by numbers" statin guidelines may consign millions of Americans to unnecessary expense and side effects for little actual benefit. On the *Today Show* one morning, I saw an interview with a medical spokesperson from the American Heart Association (AHA), noting that side effects from statins are "very rare—less than one in a thousand." This is patently false. A high percentage of patients I put on statins have to stop, most of them complaining of muscle aches. New studies also suggest subtle memory problems, particularly in older individuals, as well as the familiar liver problems. At the same time, many at-risk individuals aren't receiving the aggressive care they need.

• **Fact three:** We have a fixation with the cholesterol hypothesis when other risk factors may be at play, as well, including C-reactive protein (a marker of inflammation), homocysteine, and insulin resistance (all discussed later in this chapter).

• **Fact four:** A disconnect also exists between plaque blockage (fatty deposits) in the arteries and risk. What your cardiologist sees ("Yup, there it is—a 'widow maker'") is often only part of the story. There are really two types of plaque. "Stable plaque" has limited potential to rupture and cause a heart attack or stroke while "inflammatory plaque" (detected via blood measurements of C-reactive protein) is potentially deadly.

• **Fact five:** Reversal *is* possible with lifestyle modification and supplements—and without drugs or costly procedures. This is the essential message of breakthrough research by Dr. Dean Ornish, whose cardio programs preach diet, exercise, and meditation. In fact, many studies suggest that risk reduction via lifestyle modification can actually trump the benefits achieved

SYNDROME X

With so much focus on cholesterol we've also tended to overlook the single biggest determinant of cardiovascular risk—a constellation of hereditary (but avertable) risk factors known by several names, including metabolic syndrome, insulin resistance, and Syndrome X.

A whopping 27 percent of Americans are believed to have Syndrome X, which involves a reduced sensitivity in the tissues of the body to the action of insulin. Insulin is the hormone responsible for making sure energy, in the form of glucose, or blood sugar, finds its way into cells. Insulin resistance, or Syndrome X, means that cells respond sluggishly to the action of insulin and don't take up circulating glucose as quickly. In turn, extra glucose left in the blood signals even more insulin to be released in an attempt to prompt cells into action. It's a vicious cycle that eventually throws the body off balance—with particularly devastating results for the cardiovascular system.

Individuals with Syndrome X have at least three of five heart-disease risk factors: a top (or systolic) blood pressure reading greater than 130; a blood glucose level of 120 or more (also a risk factor for diabetes); high triglyceride levels; low levels of high-density lipoprotein or "good" cholesterol; and a large waist. Interestingly, studies show that middle-aged adults who appear to be at low risk for heart disease by standard measures, but who have Syndrome X, are also more likely to have clogged arteries that predispose them to later heart problems.

Therefore, treating cholesterol merely as an isolated phenomenon using drugs, without addressing Syndrome X, seems like a serious wrong turn in our efforts to curb America's heart-disease epidemic. The key is earlier testing (including measures of glucose tolerance with insulin, LDL and HDL cholesterol, hemoglobin A1c, and C-reactive protein), so that prevention strategies, like a heart-healthy diet and exercise, can be put into place *before* problems occur. See Chapter 4 for additional heart disease tests.

LOW-FAT OR LOW-CARB

Just what is a heart healthy diet? I have attended scores of scientific conferences on nutrition, and the debate between the low-fat and low-carb camps continues to rage without resolution. Both sides wield reams of data showing that their diet works better at helping people lose weight and alleviate cardiovascular risk. So what gives?

I've spent a lot of time thinking about this—after all, nutrition is my life's work—and it's my belief that a key factor accounts for America's diet confusion.

Genetic diversity.

One of the reasons it's hard to do studies on the "ideal diet" is that investigators are usually asking the wrong question. The answer to, "What should everyone eat?" shouldn't be "Low-fat" or "Low-carb"; it should be "Depends."

Enter the burgeoning science of "nutrigenomics," the study of how our individual genetic makeups influence what each of us should eat to maintain optimum health. At one biotechnology company, NutraGenomics, Inc., researchers even make the claim that their early research has the potential to unravel the diet conundrum.

Good news. In the meantime, though, we'll probably continue being bombarded with contradictory claims—a bewildering problem that even leads some to ignore healthy food choices altogether. "Why bother?" the thinking goes. "Next year they'll tell us to eat peat moss!"

The scientific reasons for these conflicting messages are pretty straightforward. A big one is that many studies try to link a specific diet with a particular disease in hundreds or even thousands of people. The assumption is that every person is identical. But this isn't true. Humans may share nearly the same DNA sequence (99.9 percent identical!), but it's the small (0.1 percent) differences between people that dramatically change how individuals respond to food. This also explains why some people can smoke and not develop cancer, or eat anything and not gain weight.

In other words, it's okay to use these association-studies to devise general recommendations for a population—but not for individuals. Unfortunately, we tend to use these findings as though they were one-size-fits-all. For more on genetically based nutritional approaches to disease prevention, read *Feed Your Genes Right,* by Jack Challem.

Dueling Diets

So why has neither a low-carb nor low-fat approach revolutionized health in America or stemmed our rising tide of obesity? In the 1970s, Dr. Nathan Pritikin and Michio Kushi each championed quasi-vegetarian diets with minimal fats. The government chimed in with recommendations that Americans drastically curb fat intake and the Food Pyramid was born, emphasizing generous helpings of bread and pasta, starchy vegetables, and succulent, sugary fruit. But then a strange thing happened: the percentage of adults deemed overweight soared from around 25 percent in the 1970s to nearly 70 percent in the late 1990s. Rates of childhood obesity skyrocketed.

Suddenly, the low-carb message began to resonate. Championed by Dr. Robert Atkins and Dr. Barry Sears, these new diets called for cutting carbs and loading up on protein. Many Americans briefly shed weight, before they began defecting to Weight Watchers or Jenny Craig as the pounds came back with a vengeance.

Part of the reason is that restrictive diets—whether they banish carbs, fat, or yellow and green foods on odd days of the week—help you stabilize or lose weight in the short term because they thrust a barrier between you and the refrigerator. But human ingenuity and free-market capitalism often undermine even the best intentions of most diets. Diet movements may start out pure, but most eventually get lost in translation.

I remember the macrobiotic movement, a program of strict veganism (no animal products, or dairy and eggs) that got started in the 1970s. The foods were elaborately prepared, consisting largely of big steaming pots of brown rice, root vegetables and greens, mounds of beans and tofu. But as a result of its popularity, health-food stores began sporting convenient and more palatable versions of the diet. These alternatives conformed to the rules, but made things a little more interesting—naturally sweetened, toasted brown rice snacks, mock hamburgers and hot dogs, frozen fake soy lasagna, and luscious soy- and brown-rice ice cream. Certainly these goodies rescued bored palates and helped the movement thrive, but such offerings ran contrary to the austere spirit intended by the diet's originators. American ingenuity once again imitated, co-opted, revised, and homogenized. And presto! "Lost in Translation."

A similar fate befell Dr. Dean Ornish in the 1980s. The diet he originally proposed was ultra low-fat and natural, but inadvertently spawned the marketing of low-fat Kraft Snackwells, fat-free Entenmann's pastries, and even a classic Seinfeld episode (with a cameo by then-New York Mayor Rudy Giuliani) about scrumptious low-fat "diet" frozen yogurt that, contrary to its billing, could *not* be eaten in unlimited amounts.

The same fate ultimately caught up with the late Dr. Atkins. Marketers exploited his low-carb, high-protein concept in ways that would've made him wince—devising foods that were low in "net carbs" but high in poor quality fats, artificial ingredients, and caloric sweeteners.

The "Polymeal" Diet

The search for a magic heart-healthy elixir continues—often with amusing results. A recent article in the *British Medical Journal* proposed a "Polypill" for everyone over fifty-five, consisting of three blood pressure drugs, a cholesterol-lowering statin, aspirin, and B vitamins to lower homocysteine.[1] The authors claimed it could cut cardiovascular death by a whopping 80 percent!

Needless to say, the article whipped up a firestorm of controversy among medical authorities. One of my favorite responses called for a tastier non-pill alternative, dubbed the "Polymeal."[2] Instead of five drugs and a vitamin supplement, researchers recommended feasting regularly on a combination of six heart-healthy foods (wine, fish, dark chocolate, fruits/veggies, garlic, and almonds).

I say why stop at six? Let's add green tea (helpful in reducing inflammation linked to cardiovascular risk); flaxseed (shown to reduce cholesterol, as well as cutting the risk of prostate and breast cancer); and soybeans (lower cholesterol) to this important list of heart-boosting foods!

Salad and Salmon Diet

While I customize diets to meet my patients' individual needs, I find the Salad and Salmon Diet, which I invented in the 1980s, offers some of the best heart protection around. Not only does it limit refined carbs (sugars, juices, flours, and starches), but it also emphasizes low-glycemic index carb sources, like beans and brown rice. Low-glycemic foods tend to be higher in fiber and lower in fat, resulting in a smaller rise in blood sugar and better insulin sensitivity (remember that insulin resistance, or Syndrome X, is a prime contributor to heart disease).

The Salad and Salmon Diet also encourages nuts, which are rich in vitamins and heart-healthy essential fatty acids. Fats are okay in moderation, as long as they're mostly from sources like olive, flax, or fish oil (I banned trans fats from the get-go—long before they were widely-acknowledged to be harmful!). In addition, I encourage eating protein from both vegetable and animal sources, but prefer range-fed or organic sources with plenty of fish and legumes. Abundant low-starch vegetables and moderate fruit servings provide essential fiber and protective phytonutrients (antioxidant plant compounds, including carotenoids and lignans, that boost immunity and fight free-radical damage). Using this diet, it's not unusual for patients to lose fifty pounds or more, as well as slash blood sugar, blood pressure, cholesterol, and C-reactive protein.

A-List Foods on the Salad and Salmon Menu

The Salad and Salmon Diet emphasizes lean protein, healthy fats such as olive oil and fish oil, low-glycemic index vegetables and fruits, and phytonutrient-rich legumes, nuts, and spices while minimizing starches, sugars, saturated fats, synthetic additives, and processed oils.

- **Protein:** Chicken, turkey, low-mercury containing fish (salmon and artic char are excellent choices), extra-lean sirloin, flank steak, lean pork, and eggs. Note: Free-range and organic sources of meat are preferable because they are relatively free of antibiotics and growth hormones. Best is grass-fed beef, which most closely approximates what our nineteenth-century ancestors consumed when heart disease was a rarity.

- **Eggs:** Most individuals may consume up to six eggs per week. (Quantity adjusted for each individual.) Buy organic brands.

- **Nuts and nut butters:** Almonds, Brazil nuts, cashews, filberts, macadamia, pecans, pine nuts, pistachios, and walnuts.

- **Seeds and seed butters and pastes:** Flax, pumpkin, sesame, sunflower, tahini.

- **Legumes:** Adzuki, black-eyed peas, black turtle beans, garbanzo beans (chickpeas), kidney beans, lentils, lima beans, mung beans, navy beans, peas, pinto beans, soybeans (edamame) and minimally refined soybean products, such as tempeh and tofu.

- **Fruit:** Look for organic apples, fresh or frozen berries (blueberries, raspberries, strawberries), grapefruit, oranges, and pears. Quantities are limited to two 4-ounce servings per day.

- **Non- and low-starch vegetables:** Buy organic asparagus, avocado, green/wax beans, beets and beet greens, bok choy, broccoli, Brussels sprouts, cabbage, cauliflower, celery, chard, chicory, collard greens, crookneck squash, cucumber, dandelion, eggplant, endive, escarole, kale, kohlrabi, leek, mushrooms, mustard greens, okra, onion, parsley, parsnips, radishes, romaine lettuce, rutabaga, scallions, spinach, summer squash, sprouts, Swiss chard, turnips, watercress, zucchini.

- **Sea vegetables:** Arame, dulse, hijiki, kelp, laver, nori, and wakame.

- **Whole, unprocessed grains:** Amaranth, barley, brown rice, bulgur wheat, kamut, millet, oats, quinoa, and spelt. Quantity of complex carbohydrate allowed per person is based on lab data and level of activity. The usual starting point is no more than one to two 4-ounce servings per day.

- **Oils for salads and cooking:** Extra-virgin olive oil, and cold-pressed or unprocessed avocado, flax, grapeseed, macadamia nut, peanut, and walnut oils. (Note: Flax oil, the densest vegetarian source of omega-3 fatty acids, is incredibly sensitive to heat so it's best not to cook with it.)

- **Dairy:** Yogurt (plain, Stonyfield is the best brand). Cottage cheese 1 percent, or feta cheese. Organic sources are preferable.

- **Beverages:** Water, herbal tea, and seltzer. (Try using flavored seltzers instead of soda. The brands Canada Dry and Poland Spring make great-tasting seltzers such as lemon, lime, and cherry.) Limit juice portions depending on your metabolism—overweight patients and those with insulin resistance are discouraged from juices altogether.

For more on the diet, check out www.drhoffman.com/page.cfm/21.

SUPPLEMENT PROTECTION

In addition to a good multivitamin and mineral formula, prevent heart disease with these additional supplements:

- **Carnitine:** One 500 milligrams (mg) tablet twice daily
- **Coenzyme Q_{10}:** 60–90 mg/day
- **Fish oil:** One to two 1,000 mg capsules/day
- **Kyolic (aged garlic extract):** One 1,000 mg capsule/day
- **Magnesium:** Counting the amount in your multiple, 400 mg of additional

elemental magnesium (not the weight of the pills, but the actual amount of magnesium they deliver, usually indicated on the label). My favorite sources are magnesium citrate, glycinate, or taurate (the best for arrhythmias, but the most expensive). Magnesium can have a laxative effect (welcomed by some patients). If so, be sure to ease up slowly.

• **Niacin:** 50 mg twice daily. Some people experience facial flushing, which can be prevented by taking niacin with food. Higher doses, which are very effective at lowering bad LDL cholesterol and raising good HDL cholesterol, should be taken only under a doctor's supervision because of niacin's tendency to cause liver trouble.

• **Tocotrienols:** 50–100 mg twice daily. These members of the vitamin E family are potent antioxidants that protect against hardening of the arteries.

• **Vitamin E:** 400–800 international units (IU) a day of natural mixed tocopherols (limit to 200 IU if you're over sixty-five with serious heart problems).

EXERCISE

For years, heart experts have emphasized aerobic exercise as the best road to heart health. Unfortunately, strength training has gotten lost in the shuffle. Indeed, to this day, many doctors recommend only gentle aerobics to their patients at risk for heart disease, and discourage resistance exercises like weight-lifting, for fear it puts inordinate strain on the heart.

Certainly aerobic exercises, like brisk walking, jogging, or bicycling promote circulation and optimize beneficial HDL cholesterol. They also offer a hedge against weight gain. But new findings also confirm the unique benefits of strength training and resistance exercises. Both sustain and build muscle mass, which in turn defends against Syndrome X.

Normally, when insulin is released by the pancreas it prompts muscle tissue to pull excess glucose out of the blood for use as energy or for storage. However, when muscle mass declines from lack of exercise or age (without training most of us lose about 10 percent per decade after age forty), insulin sensitivity is reduced. In turn, muscle tissues don't get the message to grab glucose and excess blood sugar and insulin build up, leading to insulin resistance, or Syndrome X. This is true even for slender individuals who don't appear at high risk for heart disease.

New studies also confirm that resistance training several times a week stokes the body's resting metabolic rate—how fast you burn calories when you're not exercising—more effectively than the same amount of aerobic exercise. (Think of those disappointing "total calories expended" scores that an hour of high-intensity pavement-pounding or cardio kickboxing actually gets you.)

Check with your doctor about the level of strength training that's right for you. For instance, if you're prone to strokes or heart attacks or have poorly controlled glaucoma, you certainly don't want to bench press your own weight. But when practiced safely (using moderate weights with more repetitions under proper supervision), weight-lifting not only regulates blood pressure, but it's also ideal for diabetics, those at risk for osteoporosis, and as a hedge against back and neck problems that occur with aging.

Since many doctors aren't up on the latest exercise recommendations, consider a medically supervised cardiac rehabilitation program at a local hospital or medical facility, particularly if you're at risk for heart problems. Also, be sure to diversify your exercise portfolio with aerobics, stretching exercises like yoga, and strength training, preferably on separate days for maximum effect. See Resources for Patients for more on strength training.

TELL YOUR CARDIOLOGIST ABOUT THESE

Whether you're trying to head off heart disease or being treated for a current heart condition, these highly promising evidenced-based therapies are ones that even a conventional doctor can embrace—or should after boning up on the research.

Coenzyme Q_{10}

I first heard about CoQ_{10} in the 1980s when I attended a lecture by the "Father of CoQ_{10}," Dr. Karl Folkers. He had just isolated a substance present in all cells (hence its scientific name *ubiquinone*) that was especially important for energy production in the body's hardest-working cells, those of the heart muscle. CoQ_{10} was said to be helpful for patients with failing heart muscle, or congestive heart failure (which may soon eclipse heart attacks as our biggest heart problem).

I began using CoQ_{10} for some of my heart patients, but initially prescribed relatively low doses until one of my patients inadvertently taught me the value of ratcheting things up a notch. At first, she had little luck easing her shortness of breath with the dose I gave her, so I suggested doubling it. After a month, her symptoms were better, but she still had difficulty making it up steep hills. Something changed during a trip to San Francisco. She returned reporting that her walking ability had improved dramatically. When I asked to see her pills, I discovered that she'd run out while on vacation and had inadvertently bought a brand containing double what I'd recommended. At 300 mg of CoQ_{10} per day she was achieving benefits that had eluded her at 150 mg.

Ironically, CoQ_{10} is depleted by virtually all statin drugs, so if you're taking one, it's more important than ever to replenish this essential nutrient. A radio listener recently wrote me with a "miracle" story about CoQ_{10} and statins. Her husband began complaining of pain and tingling in his back, leg, and arm after starting on Pravachol. Luckily, she remembered hearing on my show that these might be side effects from taking statins without CoQ_{10}. Instead of reaching for aspirin or Aleve to combat his pain, or stopping the Pravachol altogether, she purchased a bottle of 100 mg supplements, and in five days his symptoms had disappeared completely and permanently.

CoQ_{10} also benefits patients with arrhythmias, and may even lower blood pressure. Currently, it's receiving lots of attention in the field of neurology for its role in easing the symptoms of Parkinson's disease, and maybe even ALS (amyotrophic lateral sclerosis or Lou Gehrig's disease), Alzheimer's disease, and Huntington's disease (see Chapter 9 for more on cognitive and sensory problems).

Note: Your doctor may challenge your decision to take CoQ_{10} supplements. Indeed, several studies have appeared in medical journals questioning the efficacy of CoQ_{10}. But most of these were performed in an era when insufficient doses were used, and researchers believed they could put the kibosh on CoQ_{10}, once and for all. Additionally, CoQ_{10} is thought to sometimes interact with the blood thinner Coumadin, so be sure to coordinate with your doctor if you're taking Coumadin and plan to introduce CoQ_{10} (see "The Low-Down on Drug/Nutrient Interactions" on page 112).

For heart disease prevention, I recommend 60–90 mg a day. For offsetting the effects of statin drugs, try 90–150 mg daily. For congestive heart failure, arrhythmias, mitral valve prolapse, or blood pressure optimization, take 150–400 mg a day. (Ask your doctor to measure your blood levels of CoQ_{10} to see if you're achieving therapeutic levels.)

Fish Oil

Of all the cardio-protective nutrients, fish oil with its abundant omega-3 essential fatty acids (EFAs) is the most universally accepted among doctors. Indeed, more than ten years of follow-up data for more than 200,000 subjects showed a 25 percent reduction in risk of heart disease deaths when fish oil was taken at the recommended level.[3]

Studies show that fish oil's cardio benefits (whether taken in supplement form or by eating fish) are numerous. A few of these benefits include:

- Preventing blood clots by reducing the stickiness of platelets.

- Reducing inflammation of the arterial walls.

- Combating dangerous "unstable" plaque: One radio listener recently told me that her calcium plaque score, while still in the moderate range, dropped from 290 to 230 (a 12 percent decrease) after three months of taking fish-oil capsules.

- Improving cholesterol profiles, and in particular, lowering high triglycerides.

- Lowering blood pressure.

- Preventing cardiac arrhythmias and reducing the risk of sudden death from ventricular tachycardia and fibrillation.

- Reversing insulin resistance.

Note: Your doctor may warn that taking fish-oil supplements boosts your risk of hemorrhagic strokes (caused by a burst blood vessel). But studies show hemorrhagic strokes have only one-fifth the incidence of thrombotic strokes, which fish oil does prevent.

Be aware, too, that the type of fish you feast on matters. In general, fatty fish, like mackerel, lake trout, herring, sardines, albacore tuna, and salmon, are richer in omega-3s than farm-raised or white-meat fish. (See the inset "Fish Sense.") Frying fish can also destroy heart-protective EFAs. See http://circ.ahajournals.org/cgi/content/full/106/21/2747/TBL3 for the omega-3 content of various fish and supplements.[4]

And don't forget about environmental pollutants, which can concentrate in the fat cells of some fish. Studies are split on whether the heart-protective benefits of eating fish are offset by the presence of mercury. PCB (polychlorinated biphenyl) also continues to be a problem, particularly in farmed salmon raised on inexpensive PCB-laced fish meal. PCB was banned years ago for causing reproductive problems and possibly cancer, but continues to persist in the environment, particularly in muddy bottoms of estuaries and shallow coastal waters. Your best bet: organic farmed salmon grown with feeds certified to be PCB free.

For optimum cardio protection, eat two to three fish portions per week. If you prefer supplements, try one to two (1,000-mg) fish-oil capsules per day containing important omega-3s fatty acids DHA (docosahexanoic acid) and EPA (eicosapentaenoic acid).

FISH SENSE

Web resources for making safer fish choices:

- **Consumer Lab:** www.consumerlab.com. Rates fish-oil supplements, concluding that most are free of mercury and chemical contaminants.

- **Got Mercury:** www.gotmercury.org. Measure whether your mercury intake exceeds EPA limits by plugging in your weight and type of fish.

- **Seafood Choices Alliance:** www.seafoodchoices.org. Information on making environmentally friendly, safe, seafood choices, including SeaSense database, describing pros and cons of eating several types of fish.

Magnesium

Several large studies have shown that the more magnesium in your body, the lower your cardiac risk (See "Practice Tips for Doctors" on page 108 for citations to important studies). Additional studies show that magnesium deficiency plays a critical role in the development of ischemic heart disease (lack of blood flow and oxygen to the heart muscle), cardiomyopathy (inflammation of the heart muscle), certain arrhythmias, insulin resistance, diabetes, and several other heart conditions.

Note: Your physician may argue that the "mother of all magnesium studies," the ISIS-4 (Fourth International Study of Infarct Survival), didn't pan out.[5] In it, researchers gave intravenous magnesium to hospitalized patients. Not only was it found to be ineffective, but it also possibly increased the risk of death from cardiogenic shock (when the heart can't pump sufficient blood to the body). Because ISIS-4 evaluated more patients than all other magnesium studies combined, many cardiologists take the results very seriously. In fact, some have now concluded that intravenous magnesium has no place in the routine treatment of acute heart attacks.

Certainly, it's hard to go toe-to-toe with your cardiologist on technical details of a scientific study. However, you might point out that he or she is confusing apples and oranges. Magnesium for *prevention* of heart attacks and numerous other cardio problems is a far cry from emergency intravenous use during a heart attack.

Ask your doctor to test your magnesium levels, but be aware that commonly used magnesium blood screens aren't always strong enough to catch deficiencies in patients who appear "well." I recommend more precise tests, such as intracellular magnesium (measures magnesium in cells taken from inside the cheek) or ionized magnesium (measures the "active" form that isn't bound to carrier molecules in the blood). Using the latter test, I find the majority of my patients with heart problems have sub-optimal magnesium levels.

Replenishing magnesium stores is often difficult because the body has trouble holding onto magnesium. (See "Supplement Protection" on page 102 for recommended dosages.) Too much taken orally results in diarrhea, which paradoxically allows more magnesium to escape the body. Additionally, chronic stress tends to deplete magnesium (adrenaline causes the kidneys to "leak" it). Therefore, food sources, like nuts, whole grains and green, leafy vegetables are sometimes not enough. In these cases, oral supplements and some times intravenous treatments (which don't cause diarrhea since they bypass the GI tract) are necessary. Even then, it may take months for magnesium levels to improve.

For more on magnesium, read *The Miracle of Magnesium* by Carolyn Dean, M.D., N.D.

PRACTICE TIPS FOR DOCTORS

Check out these studies showing a link between magnesium deficiency and heart disease:

• National Health and Nutrition Examination Survey. National Center for Health Statistics, Centers for Disease Control: www.cdc.gov/nchs/nhanes.htm. Shows an inverse association between serum magnesium and incidence of heart disease in a ten-year follow-up.

• Atherosclerosis Risk in Communities. Collaborative Studies Coordinating Center, Department of Biostatistics, School of Public Health, University of North Carolina at Chapel Hill: www.cscc.unc.edu/aric/#. Shows an inverse association between serum magnesium and incidence of heart disease in four- to seven-year follow-ups.

• Durlach, Jean, P. Bac, M. Bara, et al. "Cardiovasoprotective Foods and Nutrients: Possible Importance of Magnesium Intake." *Magnesium Research* Vol. 12, No. 1 (1999): 57–61. Study of hospitalized cardiac patients showed 42.2 percent had low levels of magnesium.

• Purvis, John.R. and Assad Movahed. "Magnesium Disorders and Cardiovascular Diseases." *Clinical Cardiology* Vol. 15, No. 8 (August, 1992): 556–568. Links magnesium deficiency to numerous heart conditions, including arrhythmias, and finds use beneficial in treatment of cardio problems.

Meditation

For many doctors, meditation resides in the realm of New Age hooey—okay for Indian yogis and students of Eastern religion, but not suitable for scientific study. And certainly not a valid treatment for heart disease.

Yet study after study shows that daily meditation, for even a few minutes, can dramatically cut blood pressure by reducing stress, particularly in women. Spikes in blood pressure, even small spikes, can cause arteries to harden, aneurysms to form in blood vessels, and the heart to enlarge.

A recent study of one hundred-fifty African Americans (a group with the highest hypertension rate in the nation) found that meditating for twenty minutes in the morning and twenty minutes in the evening cut average systolic readings (the upper number indicating blood pressure during heart beats) by 3.1 points and diastolic readings (the lower number showing pressure between beats) by 5.7 points.[6] (Readings below 120 over 80 are considered normal. Those between 120/80 and 139/89 are labeled "prehypertension," and readings of 140/90 indicate hypertension, or high blood pressure.) The effect on the meditation group was significantly higher than those in a progressive muscle relaxation group and those in a regular health-education class.

Women showed an even greater blood pressure reduction (a 7.3 point drop in systolic and a 6.9 point drop in diastolic readings), compared to a .2 point systolic increase and a 4.7 point diastolic drop for men.

Meditation can be done in a variety of ways—and really requires trying out various approaches until you find one that's comfortable for you. My simple advice is to forget the contorted positions and exotic mantras (repeating a word or sound). Find some uninterrupted time, turn off the phones, set a timer, and lie down on a comfortable rug in a darkened, quiet room. Place your hands lightly on your abdomen and note the gentle rise and fall of your breathing. (If you're breathing through your chest muscles, you won't attain the proper level of relaxation.) Breathe slowly and rhythmically for five, ten, fifteen, then twenty minutes progressively. Focus on relaxing your muscles, locating sources of tension from head to toe. If distracting thoughts intrude, don't fight them. Instead try a visualization: Insert thoughts in large fluffy cumulus clouds and allow them to float off. (See Resources for Patients for more on hypertension and meditation.)

REVISITING CONTROVERSIES

The following therapies, though more controversial than those listed above, are nonetheless worth thinking about in some cases and should be discussed honestly with your doctor. Educating yourself and your physician can help make this discussion more productive.

B Vitamins

Studies show that high levels of the amino acid homocysteine are associated with the risk of heart attacks, stroke, blood clots, and dementia. *The Heart Revolution* by Kilmer McCully, M.D. sets forth the argument for employing folic acid, and vitamins B_6 and B_{12} to reverse circulatory problems because these vitamins help normalize homocysteine. It stands to reason that applying a nutritional prescription to high homocysteine might prevent disease, but recent studies have yielded mixed results in arterial protection.

While some test tube studies have shown protection against factors that promote heart disease, other studies have not. The most recent blow to the homocysteine hypothesis seemed to come in spring 2006 when two large-scale studies appeared in the influential *New England Journal of Medicine* (NEJM) that showed giving B vitamins to heart patients didn't reduce their risk.[7,8]

Even the researchers acknowledged puzzlement as to why the B vitamins didn't work after it was shown that high levels of homocysteine are so strongly correlated with heart attack and stroke risk. One explanation is that the studies, while large, were simply not big enough to detect small improvements in risk that may have occurred in 10 percent or fewer of patients. Another is that, like antioxidants, B vitamins might work best to prevent the advance of atherosclerosis in individuals whose arteries are still relatively healthy—both NEJM studies looked at individuals who had fairly advanced disease with diabetes or heart attacks, and it may have been beyond the scope of the B vitamins to reverse their problems over the relatively short duration of the studies (five years). An alternative explanation, of course, is that homocysteine is a marker for cardiovascular risk that B vitamins appear to lower, but without real effects on improving circulation, it's like putting a fresh coat of paint on an old broken down car. In fact, some cardiologists have gone so far as to suggest that high doses of B vitamins, while lowering homocysteine, may act as growth factors for plaque once it's gotten started.

Until these controversies are resolved, don't expect your regular physician to be a big proponent of B vitamin therapy for heart disease or stroke prevention. Even if future studies using B vitamins to prevent circulatory problems don't pan out, lowering homocysteine with B vitamins may yet prove to be beneficial: research points to relationships between high homocysteine and breast cancer, Alzheimer's disease, and even osteoporosis. Stay tuned—rarely in science do issues as complex as cardiovascular risk get put to bed with a "final" study that trumps the conclusions of all those that go before it.

Bottom-line: Ask your doctor to test you for homocysteine (see Chapter 4).

Vitamin E

In 2004, a much ballyhooed study appeared in the *Annals of Internal Medicine* warning of harmful effects from taking vitamin E supplements.[9] Vitamin E is one of several critical antioxidants, including vitamins C and A, that guard the body against damage from free radicals generated by smoking, pollution, and inflammation. Headlines screamed "Vitamin E Death Risk." Even the usually staid *Lancet* luridly exclaimed on its front page: "The prospect that vitamin pills may not only do no good but also kill their consumers is a scary speculation given the vast quantities that are used in certain communities."[10]

In my opinion, scientists succumbed to the media's infatuation with sensational headlines and over-reached the slight statistical trends of the study. In fact, this research was actually a mélange ("meta-analysis") of prior studies looking at very sick people with cancer, kidney disease, and heart conditions—and not at ordinary individuals seeking prevention. Another problem: Study participants also took synthetic vitamin E, a form less favored for its cardiovascular benefits than natural vitamin E with mixed tocopherols and tocotrienols (the active compounds). Even so, the authors sweepingly concluded that high-dose vitamin E supplements (greater than 400 IU per day) "may increase all-cause mortality and should be avoided."

The fact is, literally hundreds of studies have laid the groundwork for vitamin E's distinct antioxidant benefits, illustrating repeatedly that it promotes circulation, defends the arterial walls from free-radical damage, and staves off heart disease. So it would be premature to abandon vitamin E as a heart protector on the basis of a single study, particularly one fraught with so many methodological pitfalls. See the Council for Responsible Nutrition's website: www.crnusa.org/vitaminEis safe.html for more on the study's flaws.

Bottom-line: Natural vitamin E (400–800 IU per day of natural mixed toco-pherols) used in synergy with other antioxidants discussed in this chapter are important components of an early prevention regimen against heart disease. If you're over age sixty-five *and* have serious cardiovascular disease (particularly if you're taking multiple drugs, including blood thinners) you might want to take a conservative stance by limiting your intake of vitamin E to 200 IU a day—that is, until further studies exonerate vitamin E (as I think they will).

For further discussion of whether antioxidants, including vitamin E, interfere with statin drugs or blood thinners, like Coumadin, see "The Low-Down on Drug/Nutrient Interactions" on page 112.

Chelation

As discussed in Chapter 4, chelation therapy relies on an oral chelator to chemi-cally grip heavy metals in the body and allow them to pass harmlessly through the kidneys and into the urine. Beyond its effects on heavy metals, like lead, cadmi-um, and mercury, chelation also helps remove inappropriate accumulations of cal-cium from tissue. This is particularly helpful against heart disease because calcium often gravitates to atherosclerotic plaque in arteries, leading to narrowing and blockage. Chelation gently and gradually dissolves calcium from plaque, restoring elasticity and flow to blood vessels.

While controversial (few orthodox cardiologists support its use), several thou-sand physicians do practice chelation therapy throughout North America and the world. Many are members of the American College for Advancement in Medi-cine (www.acam.org).

In my experience, chelation has helped many patients. I've seen it reverse angina and severe claudication (pain while walking caused by arterial narrowing). It's also halted the narrowing of coronary and carotid arteries when bypass sur-gery or stenting (insertion of a wire mesh tube to prop open a recently cleared artery) either can't be performed or aren't yet necessary.

True, there are instances where chelation is an inadequate alternative to deci-

THE LOW-DOWN ON DRUG/NUTRIENT INTERACTIONS

Here are some potential interactions between conventional heart medications and supplements that you should be aware of. Be sure to discuss them with your physician.

- **Coumadin and Natural Blood Thinners**

Supplements with blood-thinning properties, like fish oil, vitamin E, CoQ_{10}, bromelain, flaxseed, ginger, garlic, and ginkgo biloba, can sometimes add to Coumadin's (warfarin) anticlotting effect, resulting in excessive or abnormal bleeding. Coumadin is generally taken to prevent dangerous stroke-causing blood clots in people with heart arrhythmias, like atrial fibrillation.

While new awareness of these interactions has prompted some doctors to ban their patients from using suspected blood-thinning supplements, I take a different tack. For one thing, not everyone is affected the same way; some people are more sensitive to supplement-Coumadin interactions than others, particularly debilitated, malnourished, or elderly individuals. Also, I believe that many of these nutraceuticals are valuable in their own right. It's precisely those individuals with heart disease who stand to benefit most from heart-healthy fish oil, vitamin E, and Alzheimer's-protective ginkgo.

Therefore, I tend to gradually ramp up doses of these supplements with patients on Coumadin. However, I insist that they continue getting their blood-clotting speed checked frequently via a test called the Protime (PT)/INR and that they give their doctor a heads-up that their Coumadin may need to be lowered accordingly. I also keep to smaller doses (fish oil less than 2 grams daily, vitamin E less than 400 IU a day) and tell patients to be consistent in their supplement intake from day to day.

Bottom-line: In my twenty-year career, I've never seen a single problem with excessive bleeding or crazy off-the-wall PT/INR results.

- **Vitamin-K Foods and Coumadin**

Vitamin K has the opposite effect on Coumadin; it neutralizes its blood-thinning effect, leaving patients at risk for blood clots. The current vogue among some nutritionists and physicians is to counsel patients on Coumadin not to eat or drink vitamin K–containing foods, like green leafy vegetables, cruciferous vegetables, and green tea. Not only is this unnecessary, it's also extremely deleterious to patients.

For one thing, these foods are all important for heart health and fighting cancer. Another point is that patients on Coumadin need a certain amount of vitamin K to prevent possible losses in bone mineral density.[11] So go ahead and enjoy those collard greens, spinach, and kale.

Good news, too, if you want the added antioxidant and heart benefits of EGCG (epigallocatechin gallate), the chief green tea polyphenol. There are now vitamin K-free supplements, but check with the manufacturer because not all supplements have this feature. Also, go easy on herbs, like alfalfa and goldenseal, which contain substantial amounts of vitamin K.

- **Antioxidants and Statin Drugs**

A 2001 study found that patients taking the antioxidants beta-carotene, vitamin E, vitamin C, and selenium, along with cholesterol-lowering Zocor (simvastatin) and niacin (vitamin B_3), had a smaller boost in HDL (high-density lipoprotein or "good") cholesterol, and a tinier reduction in heart-harming lipoprotein (a), than those taking only a simvastatin-niacin combination.[12] The conclusion: antioxidants blunt the cholesterol-cutting effect of statin drugs. An accompanying editorial even called for a halt to recommendations that antioxidants be used to prevent and treat cardiovascular disease.[13]

But even if this small study of one hundred fifty-three patients were true, and antioxidants cut the cholesterol-lowering ability of statins (far from a foregone conclusion in my mind), the argument seems disingenuous to me. There are numerous examples of conventional drug combos whose effects clash, yet they're still deemed acceptable because each medication fulfills an important role. In my opinion, the benefits of antioxidants in preventing and treating heart disease far outweigh their risks. Bottom-line: if you're taking statins don't be afraid to make antioxidants part of your cardio-support regimen. (See "Supplement Protection" on page 102 for a list of heart-healthy vitamins.)

- **Grapefruit, Statins, and Anti-Hypertensives**

Florida grapefruit growers have literally seen their market shrink with the recognition that a compound in grapefruit and grapefruit juice can cause the body to retain higher concentrations of certain heart drugs, potentially rendering them dangerous.

However, new research offers hope to heart patients on calcium channel blockers and statins who can't dispense with their grapefruit. There are grapefruit-safe drug alternatives. For instance, hypertensive patients should avoid channel blockers, but can opt for a slew of other medications of different classes, like beta and alpha blockers, diuretics, and ACE inhibitors. And while grapefruit aficionados on statins should steer clear of Zocor, Lipitor, and Crestor, they can generally use Pravachol with minimal grapefruit interaction. For a list of medications to avoid with grapefruit, visit www.druginteractioncenter.org.

Bottom-line: As with so many healthful foods and supplements, if you arm yourself with the proper knowledge, there's no need to always throw the baby out with the bathwater.

CHELATION CONSULTATION: REACHING A COMPROMISE

When Don Morgan suffered a heart attack two years ago, his cardiologist inserted a stent and advised him to lose weight and take a statin drug. However, over time, Don began to worry that he wasn't doing enough to fight plaque buildup in his arteries that might lead to another heart attack. Here, he works out a plan to try chelation therapy that both he and his cardiologist can live with.

Don: I'd like your cooperation so you can monitor my progress while I'm trying chelation.

Dr. Tilly: You know, a lot of cardiologists think it's pure snake oil. What convinces you that chelation is worth trying, or that it's even safe?

Don: I know it's not officially recognized, but I've been doing a lot of research. I noticed on the National Institutes of Health (NIH) website* that there's a large, government-sponsored study under way, focusing on patients like me who've already had heart attacks. Don't get me wrong, I appreciate your care, and the wonderful job you did putting in that stent. But I feel I need to do more to prevent a second heart attack. Your support's really important to me.

Dr. Tilly: Okay. I'll check out what they're doing at NIH, and I'll track your progress. We'll put it to the test. But I need your cooperation, too. I'll want to make sure your annual stress test is improving, and that your blood tests aren't showing any toxic effects. Plus, give me the number of the doctor you plan to do chelation with, and I'll keep her on the same page. Let's just be objective about this: if you benefit, fine; if not, promise me you'll quit. Fair?

Don: Okay—fair enough. I really appreciate you working with me.

* http://nccam.nih.gov/chelation/

sive high-tech interventions, but it remains worthy of a place among effective cardiac therapies. It's also ideal for prevention before arteries become blocked. Plus, it provides great secondary prevention after a heart attack, stroke, or as added insurance after conventional therapy. See "Chelation Consultation" above for tips on speaking with your doctor about whether it's right for you.

Hormone Replacement Therapy (HRT)

Does HRT prevent or provoke heart disease? That's the "Million Dollar Question" since the Women's Health Initiative (WHI) study found in 2002 that an alarming number of women participants on combination HRT (estrogen and progestin) suffered heart attacks and strokes—so many, in fact, that the study was prematurely concluded to protect research subjects from harm.[14] Bad news struck again in 2004 when the estrogen-only portion of the WHI study was also cut short because of a rise in stroke risk among participants. (For more on the Women's Health Initiative, visit www.nhlbi.nih.gov/whi/index.html.)

Prior to this hormone hullabaloo, estrogen (sometimes combined with progesterone) was marketed as "heart-protective." To some it made sense that "youth hormones," designed to keep women young and sexy and their bones strong, would rejuvenate their arteries, too. Indeed, early studies seemed to indicate a heart benefit.

So, why the confusion now? HRT has actually undergone several incarnations over the years. Many early studies showing a benefit used estrogen alone in women who hadn't undergone hysterectomies and didn't need progesterone to prevent uterine cancer. This led some researchers to conclude that progesterone— not estrogen—promoted heart disease in women taking the combo.

A wrinkle in that theory came in 1995 from a study called the Postmenopausal Estrogen/Progestin Interventions (PEPI) Trial, which showed heart problems in women taking *synthetic* progestogens, but not *natural* progesterone.[15]

Yet another piece of the confusion may lie in the fact that estrogen, while rejuvenating, also has a tendency to produce thickening of the blood, which can lead to blood clots. These are likely to show up as alarming upticks in heart attacks and strokes during the first few years of a trial, particularly in clot-prone women and those with the beginnings of heart disease. The result? Studies may be scuttled before long-term cardiovascular benefits can be assessed.

In fact, the "HRT for heart protection hypothesis" is not dead. More studies are planned to assess the effects of various doses of different hormone combinations. One of these, the Kronos Early Estrogen Prevention Study (KEEPS) will be particularly important in establishing once and for all whether estrogen is beneficial in preventing early lesions of atherosclerosis, but ineffective, or even harmful, once disease is established. A male version, called Testosterone Effects on Atherosclerosis in Aging Men or TEAAM Study, is also underway. See Resources for Patients for additional information on these studies.

Bottom-line: I recommend that women *not* take hormones after normal menopause unless they're suffering from severe symptoms: unmanageable hot flashes, sleep disturbances, or vaginal discomfort. Granted, more study is needed about the impact of hormones on heart health. But in the meantime we shouldn't deprive women who need menopause help from the benefits of HRT. I prescribe natural "bio-identical" estrogen and progesterone, balanced with DHEA and testosterone. I prefer formulations from compounding pharmacies that specialize in customized natural HRT therapies, such as College Pharmacy or Women's International Pharmacy (see Resources for Patients). Practitioners familiar with prescribing natural hormones may be found on the American College for Advancement in Medicine's website (www.acam.org). For more on HRT to treat symptoms of menopause and andropause, see Chapter 10.

As we've seen, heart disease isn't an inevitable part of aging. Nor is it always written in the genes. In countless cases, poor diet and lifestyle choices are at the root of heart disease. What's more, it can often be reversed with good nutritional strategies, dietary supplements, exercise and other healthy lifestyle changes— either in conjunction with conventional therapies or sometimes alone. In the next chapter, we'll see how a similar approach may also work in cancer prevention and treatment.

Cancer

Don't touch that dial
Don't try to smile
Just take this pill
It's in your file . . .
No caffeine
No protein
No booze or nicotine
Remember—
. . . Everything gives you cancer

—*CANCER* BY JOE JACKSON

Recent articles have hailed progress in the war on cancer. Experts point to statistics they say reflect rising survival rates and falling death rates from "preventable" cancers, like breast and colon. Some oncologists even envision a time when cancer will ultimately follow in the footsteps of AIDS, morphing into a treatable, chronic disease that responds to a "cocktail" of targeted drugs.

Nevertheless, cancer remains a big killer, recently surpassing heart disease as the No. 1 cause of death in Americans under eighty-five. Critics of the new-cancer optimism emphasize that seeming advances in cancer treatment may be inflated. Ralph W. Moss, Ph.D., author of *Questioning Chemotherapy* and developer of the website www.cancerdecisions.com (a leading online cancer information and referral service), points out that recent boosts in the five-year survival rate of many cancers are artifacts of "lead-time bias." That is, our ability to detect cancer very early has been vastly improved with PSAs (prostate specific antigens), mammograms, colonoscopies, PAP smears, and other sophisticated imaging techniques. Thus, patients with cancer may only *appear* to live longer because they were diagnosed earlier. Many aggressively screened and treated patients also have slow-growing, very early prostate and breast cancers that probably wouldn't curtail their life span anyway, even if left undiscovered.

Even more vociferous is Clifton Leaf, executive editor of *Fortune* magazine and himself a Hodgkin's survivor, who recently wrote: "Optimism is essential, but the percentage of Americans dying from cancer is still what it was in 1970 . . . and in 1950."[1] Leaf contends that cancer researchers have taken a simplistic approach, driven by drug companies seeking a profitable "magic bullet," and calls for changing how we think about cancer. The idea is to nip cancer in the bud well before it turns malignant and deadly.

In this chapter, we'll consider how this might be achieved. We'll look at lifestyle factors that may help prevent cancer. We'll also focus on some promising natural therapies that might disarm cancer before it causes harm and may also aid in cancer treatment. In addition, we'll sort through a few controversies that continue to swirl around certain CAM cancer therapies, plus examine questions and concerns you and your doctor may want to discuss.

LIVING RIGHT TO PREVENT CANCER

Naturally, the best approach to battling cancer is preventing it in the first place. Unfortunately, researchers still haven't devised that magic lifestyle regimen that can do the trick.

For example, many studies have examined diet's effect on the risk of developing cancer. Various links have been proposed, but the results don't agree. For instance, consumption of fruits and vegetables seems to confer protection in some studies, but others, astonishingly, refute even this tried-and-true cancer-prevention strategy. Some studies link consumption of animal fat to certain cancers, while others indict meat, especially when processed or charbroiled. Surprises also abound: For example, Italian researchers, intent on finding a link between saturated fat and breast cancer, found none at all. Instead, total carbohydrate intake seemed to boost risk, casting doubt on pasta, *biscotti,* and *zabaglione.*

Such confusion harkens back to the controversy surrounding heart disease and nutrition (see Chapter 6). Just as cardio researchers haven't yet settled upon the perfect heart-healthy diet, so cancer specialists have yet to find a nutritional course that will block cancer.

The Technicolor Diet

Though a foolproof cancer diet doesn't exist, there are some foods that seem to confer a protective effect. I recommend seeking out brightly colored fruits and vegetables from the entire color spectrum. Those bright pigments are signatures for antioxidant-rich plant compounds called phytonutrients, including carotenoids (yellow, green, orange, and red) that act in concert to inhibit tumor progression, and anthocyanidins (blue and purple), which are among nature's best cancer fighters. Eat the following foods on a daily basis or as often as you can:

• **Berries:** Rich in cancer-fighting proanthocyanidins and ellagic acid. The good news is that jams and jellies concentrate some of the benefits of fresh berries (but beware of the high sugar content).

• **Grapes:** Researchers recently identified a dozen phytonutrient compounds found in all grapes, called flavonoids, that work together to dramatically inhibit an enzyme that aids in the proliferation of cancer cells.[2]

• **Green leafy vegetables, carrots, and beets:** All are rich in carotenoids. While artificial beta-carotene turned out not to deliver consistent preventive benefits, carotenoids in their natural form protect cells from cancerous changes.

• **Tomatoes and watermelon:** One of the pigments that makes them red is lycopene, a carotenoid that seems to guard against several cancers, particularly prostate. New data suggests it may work against colon and pancreatic cancers, as well. The good news for lovers of Italian cuisine is that cooking tomatoes and adding olive oil only serves to intensify the cancer-combating impact of lycopene.

Other cancer-fighting foods to include at mealtimes:

• **Cruciferous vegetables:** Brussels sprouts, cauliflower, cabbage, and broccoli (especially newly germinated broccoli seeds) all contain useful anticancer compounds, like indole carbinols and isothiocyanates. Aim for a serving a day.

• **Flax:** With its high-lignin content (another important phytonutrient), flax seems to offer protection against hormonal cancers, like breast and prostate. It's also good for cholesterol reduction and a great hedge against constipation (a risk factor for some gastrointestinal cancers). Try 1 or 2 tablespoons of freshly ground flaxseed per day—it's great over salads or on oatmeal.

• **Onion family:** Onions, shallots, and garlic contain valuable cancer-battling compounds called polyphenols, including quercetin. It turns out the stronger and more pungent the flavor, the better the protection. Nature's trade-off: bad breath.

• **Tea:** In particular, green tea has been found to have cancer-preventive effects in large studies conducted in China. The key ingredient is apparently EGCG (epigallocatechin gallate), a polyphenol compound. EGCG seems to ward off cancer by blocking the toxicity of environmental contaminants, and by mimicking the effects of certain commonly used chemotherapy agents. The Stash brand is one of the best green teas on the market with one of the highest concentrations of protective polyphenols.

Exercise and Alcohol

The word isn't completely out yet, but many studies show that exercise is an important hedge against cancer, and can even help prevent its recurrence. Hence, those cancer walks held across the country to raise funds and awareness may actually bestow health benefits to survivors, as well. It's not clear exactly how exercise fights cancer. One theory suggests that it boosts insulin metabolism (discussed later in this chapter). Another hypothesizes that it may moderate excess levels of cancer-promoting sex hormones, like estrogen. Still others suggest that it enhances immunity or even provides more oxygen to tissues (lack of oxygen in cells is believed to foster cancer growth). It's a fair bet, then, that along with heart benefits, adopting a fitness regimen will give you some cancer protection, as well.

Moderate drinking offers some heart benefits, but when it comes to cancer, the plot thickens. We know that among alcoholics, especially those who smoke, cancer rates soar. And studies show that as few as two or three drinks per week increase women's risk for breast cancer. The reason is that even moderate consumption of alcohol robs the liver of some of its estrogen-metabolizing efficiency, thus exposing some drinking women to a higher risk of hormonal cancers.

CHEMOPREVENTION

While it might sound far-fetched that medical science may soon head off cancer in its earliest stages before it turns lethal, think of what we're doing to curb heart disease in this country. Patients are being aggressively screened for risk factors—diabetes, hypertension, high cholesterol—and remedial action is being undertaken *before* the disease advances.

The idea behind chemoprevention is similar. Tumors (like heart attacks) aren't the first sign of disease. Both are the result of accumulated genetic and environmental processes that may take years to manifest as a full-blown disease. Researchers increasingly believe that these and other diseases of aging may be linked by common pathways, such as inflammation, that can be disrupted by taking a daily pill or other therapy.

Toward this end, a wide array of natural and designer compounds are currently being investigated for their potential to prevent cancer, augment standard treatments, or prevent cancer's recurrence. A leader in this area is the University of Texas M.D. Anderson Cancer Center. Researchers there have begun identifying preventive therapies for people who are genetically at risk. These include retinoids (compounds related to vitamin A); the green tea phytonutrient EGCG; nonsteroidal anti-inflammatory drugs; curcumin (one of the main spices in curry); and selective estrogen receptor modulators (SERMs), such as raloxifene (Evista) and tamoxifen (Nolvadex), which occupy estrogen-receptor sites and block the body's own harmful estrogens from promoting cancer.

TELL YOUR ONCOLOGIST ABOUT THESE

Few conventional doctors can refute the promise these natural therapies hold for preventing and treating cancer.

Fish Oil

With its omega-3 fatty acids (good fats), such as EPA (eicosapentaenoic acid), fish oil earned high marks in the previous chapter on heart disease, and it deserves a place of prominence here, too. And as in heart disease, it has a multitude of synergistic cancer-fighting actions:

- **Combats inflammation.** Colon cancer is thought to be caused, at least in part, by chronic inflammation, since its incidence is hiked in patients suffering from inflammatory bowel diseases, like ulcerative colitis and Crohn's disease. Other examples include lung cancer and smoking (which causes inflammation), as well as esophageal cancer and chronic gastroesophageal reflux (also an inflammatory condition). Fish oil's anti-inflammatory effects extend not just to the blood vessels, or the joints, but are also pervasive throughout the body.

- **Reduces insulin resistance.** Fish oil is one of the most effective ways to sensitize the cells' insulin receptors (see next page).

- **Favorably alters gene expression.** Fish oil helps regulate mechanisms for proper cell growth, preventing out-of-control proliferation and the spread of tumors.

- **Slows cancer-wasting (cachexia).** After cancer has developed, fish oil slows the wasting away of patients' bodies by blocking a compound called tumor necrosis factor, an immune-system peptide that destroys healthy cells when levels are elevated.

At least a dozen studies show that fish oil has a protective effect against colon, breast, and prostate cancers. And while not all epidemiological studies agree, recent research looking at fish oil's relationship to lung cancer in Japanese subjects found that both men and women who ate cooked or raw fish five times a week or more had half the incidence of lung adenocarcinoma when compared to participants who ate cooked or raw fish less than once a week.[3]

A word of warning: While omega-3 fatty acids, like EPA, seem to be beneficial, an excess of omega-6 oils from refined vegetable fats (commonly used for frying) appear to boost cancer risk. Additionally, hydrogenated trans fats from margarine and shortening, or those used in commercial fast-food fryers, are also likely carcinogenic. Thankfully, their use is finally being phased out of snack foods, and eventually should disappear from eateries.

Supplementing with fish oil has a place in both prevention and treatment of cancer. Note: if you're having cancer surgery or a biopsy, tell your doctor you're taking fish oil. Because of its blood-thinning properties, he or she may ask you to discontinue using it for a couple of weeks beforehand and a week or so afterward, to avoid bleeding complications. See Chapter 11 for more on preparing for surgery.

To prevent cancer, take two 1,000-milligram (mg) capsules of fish oil with EPA/DHA daily. For treatment, take four to six capsules per day as tolerated (some patients may experience nausea, especially if they're undergoing chemo). A packet or two a day of a tasty, custard-like emulsified fish oil, called Coromega, provides an alternative for some finicky patients. See Chapter 6 for more on choosing the best fish-oil supplements and fish foods.

Insulin Resistance and Cancer

Insulin resistance, or Syndrome X, which played such an important role in our discussion of heart disease in the previous chapter, may also be a culprit in cancer. Remember that insulin resistance is reduced sensitivity in the tissues to the action of insulin, whose job it is to bring glucose in for energy. In turn, the body overcompensates by secreting more insulin from the pancreas, which eventually can result in high blood pressure, high blood glucose, elevated triglycerides, low levels of high-density lipoprotein or "good" cholesterol, and extra pounds (particularly around the waist).

Studies clearly show a higher cancer rate in overweight people. Type 2 diabetics, who are awash in excess insulin, also have far higher risk of malignancy, particularly gastrointestinal and reproductive cancers.

Insulin resistance seems to encourage cancers in several ways. One is by simply providing too much nutrition to cells—including fast-growing cancer cells. Another is by hiking levels of cancer-promoting estrogen (engorged fat cells act as tiny estrogen factories). On top of that, high insulin levels at cell-receptor sites, particularly in the colon and breast, seem to promote growth of pre-cancerous cells. In addition, the excess pounds that are a hallmark of insulin resistance may signify overconsumption of unhealthy foods laced with environmental carcinogens that are retained in fat cells. And, finally, insulin resistance seems to encourage chronic inflammation.

The solution? Follow my heart-healthy Salad and Salmon Diet, which may offer substantial additional protection against cancer. (For more on the diet, check out www.drhoffman.com/page.cfm/21.) Also, ramp up your exercise routine, which makes cells more responsive to insulin. Finally, take nutrients, like fish oil and vitamin D, both of which help curb insulin resistance.

Phytonutrient Supplements

In addition to eating plenty of the cancer-fighting foods listed earlier, talk to your doctor about incorporating these antioxidant-rich, plant-based supplements into your cancer-prevention or treatment regimen:

• **Curcumin:** This derivative of the kitchen herb turmeric, used in curry, is available as a standardized supplement. Take one 500-mg capsule twice daily.

• **EGCG:** While drinking green tea can confer some benefits, more aggressive prevention and cancer treatment calls for a harder-hitting supplement. I use EGCG Ultra, which delivers 70 percent polyphenol content. Just one 500 mg capsule is equivalent to sixteen cups of high-quality Stash tea (or twenty-two to fifty cups of ordinary green teas). Additionally, caffeine and vitamin K have been removed. For prevention, I recommend one capsule twice daily—for active cancer, four to six capsules per day.

• **Lycopene:** Controversy exists over whether capsules of this tomato extract deliver benefits comparable to those of real tomatoes. Nevertheless, I make use of a product called Lycomato, a functional food extract derived from tomatoes specially bred for enhanced lycopene content. Take one 500-mg capsule twice daily.

• **Zyflamend or PhytoGuard:** These standardized combination products contain several beneficial herbs that work synergistically to both ward off and treat cancer.

Zyflamend contains curcumin, green tea, ginger, oregano, rosemary, and other inflammation-fighting and cancer-preventive herbs. It's currently under study at Columbia Presbyterian Hospital for its effects on prostate cancer. Take one twice daily for prevention, two twice daily for cancer.

PhytoGuard contains green tea, broccoli extract, curcumin, quercetin, and additional phytonutrients valued for heart-protective and cancer-preventive effects. Take one twice daily for prevention, four to six daily for cancer.

Selenium

A 1996 study at the University of Arizona Medical School confirmed the dramatic cancer-preventive effects of this trace mineral.[4] Participants who took 200 mcg (micrograms) of selenium a day cut their risk of colon, prostate, and lung cancer by half. I recommend the same daily dose of selenium methionate. Food sources include Brazil nuts and fish.

Vitamin D

One of the most riveting new stories on the cancer front involves the vitamin D connection. Interest in the possibility that vitamin D deficiency and cancer are linked first arose in the 1980s when Dr. Cedric Garland of the University of California at San Diego noticed that colon cancer was more a disease of temperate climates, north and south of the equator, where sun exposure is less during the winter months. Similar trends were seen for osteoporosis and multiple sclerosis.

This led to the theory that time in the sun offers protection against these diseases. It also led cancer researchers to vitamin D (long believed to mainly strengthen bone), since it's made in the skin in response to sun exposure. Subsequent studies have confirmed correlations between adequate levels of vitamin D and protection from prostate, breast, colon, and skin cancer.

A recent melanoma study even revealed a surprising paradox: Survivors of this potentially deadly skin cancer, which may be initiated by overexposure to the sun early in life, *survived longer with additional sun exposure.*

Many doctors warn patients against sunning themselves because of cancer risk, and are uncomfortable prescribing higher than minimal doses of vitamin D, due to its known risks of calcium overload and kidney stones. However, patients can easily be tested for vitamin D with a test called 25-hydroxy D. When I supplement cancer patients with vitamin D, I aim for high-normal values and test frequently (every six weeks or so to see whether I might be undershooting or overshooting the mark).

Like many complementary physicians, I recommend natural vitamin D_3 (cholecalciferol) at doses up to 4,000–5,000 international units (IU) per day (as opposed to multivitamins and calcium combination products, which typically contain no more than 400–800 IU of vitamin D). See Resources for Patients for more on vitamin D and cancer.

REVISITING CONTROVERSIES

The following questions are worth discussing with your doctor. (See the list of "Do's and Don'ts of Open Dialogue" on page 125 for tips on discussing a holistic approach to cancer treatment.)

Does Diet Matter Once You've Got Cancer?

Since researchers can't agree on a cancer-prevention diet, it's small wonder there's no agreement on what to tell patients *after* they've developed cancer.

One thing I've noticed is that a cancer diagnosis is so terrifying to most patients it's almost as if they're bargaining with God. They will submit to radical surgery, harsh radiation, debilitating chemotherapy, and for good measure, quaff handfuls of supplements, and subsist on a diet of turnips and parsley, if they feel it will purge them of their disease. But is it a good idea to embark on a highly restricted or extreme diet once you have a cancer and are undergoing conventional therapy?

Despite the appeal of atoning for past dietary sins with a radical "cancer-busting" diet (even if one existed), there are several reasons not to go overboard after you've developed cancer. For one, chemo and radiation are designed to catch cancer cells in the act of replicating—the time when they're most vulnerable. Theoretically, then, restricting the growth (replication) of cancer cells via the "perfect" diet might actually cause them to remain static and resist treatment.

Another obstacle to observing strict dietary guidelines is that harsh cancer treatments tend to reduce appetite and render taste buds finicky. Healthy foods like broccoli, salads, and whole grains may taste unpleasant, and patients often begin gravitating toward "comfort foods" like ice cream. I sometimes surprise cancer patients going through arduous treatments by giving them a free pass on diet (though I recommend going easy on chemical additives and trans fats).

DO'S AND DON'TS OF OPEN DIALOGUE

The key to successfully combining conventional and natural cancer therapies is being honest with your doctor. Here are some tips for keeping the communication lines open:

• **DO** bring in a list of all the supplements you're taking. Or bring in the actual supplements.

• **DO** explain why you're taking them, including copies of original studies that support their use. (See Chapter 3 for more on evaluating the validity of scientific evidence.)

• **DO** provide names and numbers of any alternative practitioners you're seeing and encourage your doctor to coordinate with them on your care.

• **DO** talk about your diet, including any special nutritional approaches you're trying.

• **DO** discuss your fears, depression, and feelings of isolation.

• **DON'T** forget to mention herbal teas or any other nutritional remedy you're using, even if it seems harmless.

• **DON'T** overwhelm your doctor with too much information. A neat, orderly presentation helps, so put all studies and data in a binder or notebook. Stay away from clippings out of newspapers or popular magazines that may be sensationalized or inaccurate.

• **DON'T** try unsupported alternative therapies without first discussing the pros and cons with your doctor.

• **DON'T** be afraid to let your doctor know about any changes in your appetite, including not being hungry or craving only "comfort" foods, like mashed potatoes and ice cream.

• **DON'T** shy away from getting psychological and social help that can help boost your ability to heal.

Finally, skimpy diets accelerate the immune-suppression that occurs with cancer treatments. Not only does this encourage cancer recurrence, but it also makes patients more susceptible to complications, like infections.

Research tends to substantiate me on my thinking about diet and cancer. In one of the few studies of its kind, researchers showed that ultra low-fat, low-protein, or calorically deficient diets were associated with poorer outcomes.[5]

By the same token, dietary excess is also detrimental. This was dramatically illustrated to me when I was a medical student and signed up for a cancer-nutrition elective at Memorial Sloan Kettering Hospital in New York. At that time, doctors believed that aggressive nutritional support with feeding tubes and intravenous lines would stave off the wasting away and starvation that most cancer patients experience at the end. I was on hand when, to the dismay of researchers, the cancers actually drew on the added calories, protein, sugar, fat, and vitamins (called nutrient theft) and grew at astonishing rates, killing patients even faster.

Does this mean that diet doesn't matter at all once you've got cancer? Studies looking at the effects of saturated fat or fruits and vegetables on pre-existing cancer are only now underway, but early evidence suggests that a good diet may be beneficial during chemo and radiation. As we'll see later in "Drug-Nutrient Interactions," kids who received an antioxidant-enriched diet while getting chemo for childhood leukemia did better with fewer side effects from treatment.

And in a recent study of colon cancer, patients receiving radiation treatment with nutritional counseling and support did better than patients who either got special nutrient shakes with no dietary advice or got no nutritional support at all.[6]

I also think it's reasonable to conclude that once conventional therapies have fought cancer to a standstill, an optimal diet offers at least the same protection that it does prior to a cancer diagnosis (see above for cancer-preventive foods and supplements). In other words, once patients are done with chemo and/or radiation, I tell them to eat as if every morsel of food mattered. Each meal is either an opportunity squandered or a new chance to saturate the body in beneficial phytonutrients that prevent cancer.

Does Soy Prevent or Promote Cancer?

Few cancer controversies rage as fiercely as the one between foes and advocates of soy. This showdown first came to my attention almost twenty years ago when I spoke at a conference on women's health. I was the sole complementary physician on a panel with several conventional gynecologists, and after extolling the preventive virtues of soy and other "nutraceuticals," I was bushwhacked by one of the panelists. In her opinion, soy was estrogenic and could strengthen cancers. Needless to say, the audience left perplexed about the safety of this popular food.

I found my colleague's pronouncements on soy somewhat disingenuous, especially since her position at the time, like most doctors, was that estrogen was a boon to nearly all menopausal women. How could she promote estrogen, while nay-saying soy?

Little has changed in nearly two decades. The essential problem is that test-tube evidence often contradicts epidemiological evidence. We know, for example, that populations, like those in Asia, which consume lots of soy products from infancy, have a lower rate of breast and uterine cancer (as well as prostate cancer in men). However, some studies have shown that when breast cancer cells are grown in the presence of isoflavones, estrogenic chemicals found in soy, they proliferate more rapidly. Unfortunately, no large-scale trials have yet looked at whether women or men who consume soy have higher or lower rates of cancer. Not too surprising considering we haven't yet figured out whether estrogen therapy is advantageous—despite the millions of research dollars allocated to studying it.

The key, in my opinion, is to recognize that use of soy in traditional societies is lifelong. Current thinking is that the seeds of breast cancer (and perhaps prostate cancer) are planted early, in adolescence when the breasts begin development, or even earlier, in childhood or possibly in utero. Therefore, dietary soy may be most beneficial early in life. Middle-aged Americans' tendency to belatedly "get religion" when it comes to diet may actually undermine soy's benefits.

On the other hand, while soy has sometimes proved estrogenic in the test tube, this doesn't mean that it can't prevent cancer. Many of the drugs we use to enhance bone density (raloxifene) or prevent cancer recurrence (tamoxifen) are estrogenic SERMs.

Additionally, natural unrefined soy products contain other helpful compounds called angiogenesis blockers that prevent cancer in entirely different ways by halting a key step in cancer transformation. This may account for some studies showing that soy reduces the incidence of cancers not traditionally considered hormonal, like colon cancer.

Bottom-line: Soy can be safely enjoyed by anyone who doesn't have allergies or indigestion, unless they're recovering from breast cancer or are at high risk. And while modest intake of soy for infants and children is optional, excess intake to the exclusion of other protein sources should be avoided until we have more data.

I prefer food sources and don't recommend soy supplements, except to men recovering from prostate cancer. The best, least-refined sources are cooked soybeans (edamame), tofu, and tempeh. I recommend two to three 4–6 ounce servings of these foods per week. While soymilk is fine, it should be consumed in moderation (it's generally sweetened). The same goes for texturized vegetable protein, or TVP, which is highly refined and bereft of cancer-preventive nutrients.

THE LOW-DOWN ON
DRUG/NUTRIENT INTERACTIONS

Perhaps the most bitter paradigm clash in cancer treatment today is whether using antioxidant vitamins, minerals, herbs, and nutraceuticals helps or hinders conventional chemo and radiation therapies.

In his book *Complementary Cancer Therapies,* naturopath Dan Labriola articulates the conservative view that patients and holistic physicians often encounter with conventional doctors:

> Many non-conventional therapies have actions that are exactly the opposite of those of certain conventional treatments and can potentially interfere with the conventional treatment's ability to destroy the maximum number of tumor cells . . . the short-term result, from months to five years or more, might look better because of the positive effects of the non-conventional treatment. Over the long-term, however, the additional remaining cells left over from the interfered-with treatment could result in a recurrence.[7]

- **Antioxidants + Chemo & Radiation:** So are antioxidants beneficial or not? Dr. Kara M. Kelly, an associate professor of pediatric oncology at Columbia University, and her colleagues recently decided to find out.[8] The researchers measured blood levels of vitamins A, E, and C in 103 kids undergoing chemotherapy for the most common form of childhood leukemia, acute lymphoblastic leukemia (ALL). Blood samples were taken at diagnosis, after initial treatment, and again after treatments were stepped up.

What they found was that during therapy free-radical damage rose and antioxidant levels dipped. They also found that kids who were deficient in antioxidants had more chemotherapy side effects, and those with higher concentrations of vitamins A and E and total carotenoids had better outcomes with fewer infections and toxicity.

Even so, Dr. Kelly and her colleagues stopped short of recommending antioxidant supplements for young oncology patients. Their reason: lingering fear that supplements would interfere with treatment. However, they did advocate an antioxidant-rich diet.

Is this theoretical concern really borne out in the research? In one recent study of lung cancer patients given high-dose chemo with Taxol and carboplatin half the patients received an aggressive round of antioxidant supplements, including over 6 grams of vitamin C each day, over 1,000 IU of E per day, 25,000 IU of beta-carotene, plus selenium, copper, and zinc.[9] Ultimately, there was no reduction in the chemo's effectiveness; in fact, the antioxidant group responded slightly better to treatment and survived slightly longer than those given chemo alone (though the effect wasn't statistically significant). The authors concluded that current fears about antioxidants protecting cancer cells and blunting chemotherapy weren't substantiated. Indeed, only three studies out of dozens have ever shown antioxidants to diminish the effect of chemo or radiation.[10] The vast majority have shown either an enhanced or neutral effect.

- **Ban on Herbs:** Ultimately, this clash of paradigms puts patients in a bind. Remember my example in Chapter 2 of a beleaguered patient who was told not to take supplements by her oncologist at a well-known cancer center.

In fact, it's the policy at many leading cancer centers to reject *all* herbal remedies—regardless of quality control or research—because there's no federal oversight of supplements. The only exceptions are when a particular remedy is under study.

I think this is the height of *hubris,* especially in an era when many conventional cancer therapies remain only marginally effective, or even downright dangerous. Fortunately, a few progressive cancer hospitals, while cautious, maintain a more enlightened policy. Some, such as the Cancer Treatment Centers of America (www.cancercenter.com), even encourage the use of supplementary nutrients and herbs alongside conventional therapies.

Far preferable, but more time-consuming for doctors (and less certain than an all-out ban), is to consider each supplement on a case-by-case basis. With new web-based resources, looking up the available information is far less daunting than in the past when it took a trip to the medical library "stacks" to dust off old volumes or squint at microfiche for answers.

For example, my colleague Leo Galland, M.D., has created user-friendly software, called the Drug-Nutrient Workshop (www.nutritionworkshop.com), which allows medical practitioners to view documented or hypothetical reactions that might occur when drugs are combined with herbs, vitamins and minerals, or other supplements. As often as not, the results of such combinations with cancer drugs are not harmful. On the contrary, they protect the patient or enhance the drugs' cancer-fighting abilities. (See "Practice Tips for Doctors" on page 130 for suggestions on talking to patients about supplements and possible interactions.)

Vitamin C

In the 1980s, supposedly definitive studies performed by physician Charles Moertel at the Mayo Clinic were thought to forever debunk the theory that vitamin C could help cancer patients. Nonetheless, complementary physicians like myself, taking our cue from nutrition pioneers like Linus Pauling, Ph.D., Ewan Cameron, M.D., and Hugh Riordan, M.D., have been using *intravenous* vitamin C in our cancer patients, some of whom have outlived their initially gloomy prognoses. While no panacea, a high test-tube concentration of vitamin C inhibits the multiplication of cancer cells and, at sufficient doses, may cause them to self-destruct. See www.doctoryourself.com/riordan2.html (patients) and www.medpagetoday.com/HematologyOncology/OtherCancers/tb/2938 (doctors) for new clinical evidence that suggests vitamin C may have benefit.

Mark Levine, M.D., a vitamin C researcher at the National Institutes of Health,

---

PRACTICE TIPS FOR DOCTORS:
DISCUSSING DRUG-NUTRIENT INTERACTIONS

Oncologist Dr. Helen Siegel is treating Jeremy Richards for prostate cancer. During a recent office visit, Jeremy mentions that he's taking several nutritional supplements that he read might help beat cancer, including two powerful antioxidants pycnogenol and alpha-lipoic acid, as well as the amino acid lysine. Many of Dr. Siegel's colleagues oppose use of *all* supplements during cancer treatment for fear of adverse interactions, but she likes to take each patient's individual needs and desires into account. She asks Jerry to bring in all the supplements he's taking so she can check them out. Here are some respectful yet necessary questions that all doctors should ask to better understand their patients' health goals and help make them happen:

- Do you know what you're trying to achieve with each of these?

- Do you remember where you read about them or have copies of the studies?

- I haven't looked into possible interactions between these supplements and your regular treatment. Do you mind if we investigate this together using one of the new software programs, like the Drug-Nutrient Workshop?

- If we find anything potentially dangerous will you promise that we can discuss it and try to arrive at a workable treatment plan?

- Are there any other remedies or special foods you're eating that I should know about?

MIND-BODY THERAPIES TO EASE CANCER PAIN

With many non-drug treatments like relaxation, biofeedback, imagery, hypnosis, and acupuncture, patients find they can lower their dose of conventional painkillers or stop taking them altogether.

Ask your doctor about using one of these evidence-based methods or contact the National Center for Complementary and Alternative Medicine Clearinghouse at 888-644-6226 or nccamc@altmed-info.org to find a practitioner near you. Try this imagery exercise, called Ball of Energy (excerpted from the March 2005 Supplement to *Alternative Medicine Alert*):[11]

- Close your eyes. Breathe slowly and comfortably from your abdomen, and feel yourself relax.

- As you breathe in, say silently and slowly to yourself, "In, one, two." As you breathe out, say "Out, one, two." Breathe in this slow rhythm for a few minutes.

- Imagine a ball of healing energy forming in your lungs or on your chest. It may be like a white light. Envision it forming, taking shape.

- When you're ready, imagine that the air you breathe blows this healing ball of energy to the area of your pain. Once there, the ball heals and relaxes you.

- When you breathe out, imagine the air blows the ball away from your body. As it goes, the ball takes your pain with it.

- Repeat the last two steps each time you breathe in and out.

- You may imagine that the ball gets bigger and bigger as it takes more and more discomfort away from your body.

- To end the imagery, count slowly to three, breathe in deeply, open your eyes, and say silently to yourself, "I feel alert and relaxed." Begin by moving about slowly.

has argued that renewed research on the role of vitamin C in cancer treatment is warranted. He writes: "Only *intravenous* administration of vitamin C produces high plasma and urine concentrations that might have antitumor activity. Because efficacy of vitamin C treatment cannot be judged from clinical trials that use only oral dosing, the role of vitamin C in cancer treatment should be reevaluated."[12]

That research is now underway, and the pooled experiences of thousands of complementary doctors who have administered vitamin C intravenously for cancer is being reviewed more seriously to see if this treatment has merit.

Is There a "Cancer Personality"?

Much has been made of the link between repressed anger or exaggerated nice-ness and getting cancer. The notion that cancer sufferers essentially "grow" their own tumors from the ashes of dead-ended emotions was most famously explored by writer Susan Sontag after her own diagnosis with advanced breast cancer in 1976. Sontag, who died in December 2004, lived well beyond the five years she was given, but the controversies she plumbed in her essay *Illness as Metaphor* (namely, whether cancer might simply be just a capricious disease and not a phys-ical manifestation of repressed nature) continue to this day.[13]

Is there a "Type C," or cancer-prone personality? A recent review of the sci-entific literature suggests there may be something to the theory.[14] For instance, many studies show that psychological stress hinders the immune system's cancer-fighting natural killer (NK) cells. Depression and distress may also be linked to the development of cancer. Both are known to hamper the body's ability to repair damaged DNA and may interfere with normal programmed cell death—two pieces of the cancer puzzle.

Conversely, other studies show that psychological counseling, mind-body coping techniques, and social support enhance immune function and boost longevity among cancer patients. (For mind-body therapies that help ease cancer pain, see page 131.)

However, many studies show no evidence of any link between a person's per-sonality style and getting cancer. Recent research, for example, found no elevated cancer risk among people with either an extroverted (risk-taking personality) or a neurotic (worrying) personality.[15]

While it's a shame that mind-body theories might lead people who get can-cer to feel stigmatized ("I had a bad attitude"), they still might play an important role in prevention and recovery from cancer. It may be too simplistic to suggest there's an easily profileable "cancer personality," but constant worry and stress clearly erode the immune system, and at best subvert a person's resolve to follow a healthy lifestyle. Certainly, positive thinking has a lot to recommend it, includ-ing minimal side effects. After all, nobody ever died from thinking good thoughts.

As research continues to piece together the cancer puzzle, we learn increas-ingly that nutritional approaches and other CAM strategies can go a long way toward preventing cancer. Holistic approaches may also be effective in treating cancer. Doctors and patients alike need to pay attention to this research and begin incorporating new findings into their cancer-healing plans.

As we'll see in the next chapter on arthritis, CAM approaches often require patience and a certain amount of faith, but used in conjunction with convention-al therapies or alone can go a long way toward boosting outcomes and minimiz-ing side effects.

Arthritic
Diseases

8

We could stop the hurtin' for awhile.

—CHICAGO

In the mid-1990s I attended an exhaustive, one-week seminar on advances in internal medicine, my original field of specialization. In a series of grueling lectures, we covered cardiology, endocrinology, oncology, and finally arrived at arthritis.

There, I learned for the first time about COX-2 inhibitors for relieving the pain of rheumatoid arthritis, osteoarthritis, and exercise injuries. I remember how enthusiastic the rheumatology instructors were as they touted these new "super-painkilling drugs." COX-2 inhibitors, like Vioxx, Celebrex, and later Bextra, were designed to avoid gastrointestinal bleeding caused by older NSAIDs (non-steroidal anti-inflammatory drugs), including ibuprofen, naprosyn, and aspirin, which result in about 60,000 hospitalizations a year.

I knew about these problems firsthand, including my initial encounter with NSAID bleeding during the hot July of 1983 when I began my internship at Manhattan VA Hospital. One Sunday night, a robust fortyish African American—a typical "GI bleeder"—was admitted with severe internal bleeding. I quickly learned to force an NG (nasogastric) tube down his throat to suction out blood, all the while rushing back and forth to the blood bank for bag after interminable bag of freshly defrosted blood.

His wife said he'd begun experiencing back pain after long hours crouching on an electrical job. He started popping Advil every four hours, but after several days became nauseated. Instead of halting the medication, though, he stopped eating for a day, which only added to the Advil's corrosive effect on his stomach lining. On Sunday morning, he felt woozy during church and went home. Later, he began vomiting dark, coffee-colored blood clots. That's when his family dialed 911.

Unfortunately, the blood transfusion didn't end his woes. While recuperating in the hospital, my patient's eyes began turning yellow, and his urine became dark—a sign of hepatitis C (in those days blood for transfusions wasn't tested for the virus). The patient languished in the hospital for several more weeks. By the time he went home, he'd lost seventy pounds, and was weak and gaunt—all from an "innocent" over-the-counter (OTC) remedy used by millions for their aches and pains.

No wonder my colleagues at the seminar were so excited about COX-2 inhibitors. They arrived on the market shortly afterward and were quickly embraced by doctors and patients, racking up millions in sales. But cracks soon appeared. Many patients reported little additional benefit from the expensive pills. My own eighty-year-old mother, a rheumatoid arthritis sufferer, tried Vioxx on her doctor's recommendation, but said she preferred her daily regimen of a few aspirin. A confirmed contrarian, in retrospect she may have done herself a favor.

In September 2004, Merck & Co. pulled Vioxx from the market when evidence suggested a link to increased risk of heart attacks, blood clots, and stroke. Pfizer's Celebrex remains on the market with a new warning label about elevated cardiovascular risk. However, it agreed to suspend sales of Bextra until further talks with the Food and Drug Administration.

There's additional bad news about COX-2 inhibitors and other NSAIDs. Not only can they be dangerous, but also studies now suggest they may offer only meager, short-term pain relief.[1]

In light of this debacle, the use of alternative arthritis and orthopedic therapies doesn't sound so far-fetched. Certainly more doctors should discuss them with patients (see "Practice Tips for Doctors" below to learn what arthritis patients want most from physicians). In this chapter we'll examine ways to head off arthritic diseases, as well as orthopedic injuries. We'll also look at effective CAM therapies that you and your doctor should consider. Plus, we'll sort through

---

PRACTICE TIPS FOR DOCTORS: TELL-ALL MEDICINE

What do RA patients want from their doctors? Information—and lots of it. In a new study of six hundred adults with RA, participants' No. 1 desire was that their doctors volunteer all information about the disease's progression, medication side effects, and lab tests without being asked.[2] More than 20 percent said they felt their doctor hadn't told them enough. Women were more interested in hearing all their options than men.

Interestingly, patients' need-to-know didn't correspond to a desire for more authority in making treatment decisions. About 75 percent of participants agreed that doctors should take charge of treatment plans, particularly as RA gets worse.

current prevention and treatment controversies and examine drug-nutrient inter-actions—both good and bad.

BOOMERITIS

Baby boomers have always enjoyed life "in the fast lane," pressing themselves to stay healthier, exercise harder and hang onto youth longer than any previous gen-eration. In their drive to push the envelope, though, they've also debuted an entirely new medical phenomenon I like to call "boomeritis." Indeed, it's some-thing I know a bit about myself. I ran my first marathon at age thirty-nine, and am still competing in triathlons at fifty-three. For boomers like me, punishing daily exercise regimens take an obvious toll in terms of sports injuries. In fact, boomeritis has helped spawn a multibillion dollar sports-medicine industry.

Begun in the 1970s, the orthopedics revolution correlated with a rise in super-sized salaries for professional athletes. Bigger athletes (from improved steroids and better strength training) meant more injuries—as well as the devel-opment of innovative arthroscopic surgery to reconstruct frayed joints and extend athletes' careers. It wasn't long before these techniques found their way to a ready population of over-the-hill weekend warriors.

Lost that 100 mph overhead serve? Can't complete your daily five-mile jog? Got knee pain from those black diamond ski runs at Aspen? No problem: mod-ern orthopedics will get you moving again.

Trouble is, radical orthopedic surgery may work wonders to extend the careers of young athletes, but it doesn't always translate to the more prosaic dis-comforts of ailing golfers. In my opinion, high-tech surgery is overrated as an everyday performance enhancer; there's no orthopedic equivalent of Viagra.

Indeed, research shows that therapeutic exercises may be superior to sur-gery. Of eighty-four patients in a recent study with torn shoulder rotator cuffs, half got arthroscopic surgery, and half were enrolled in physical therapy for a year. The exercisers actually got slightly bigger benefits than those who underwent arthroscopy.[3]

Another promising non-invasive treatment, Extracorporeal Shock Wave Ther-apy (ESWT)—based on the ultrasonic stone-smashing technology used to blast kidney stones—has also proven effective in treating chronic pain linked to plan-tar fasciitis, heel spurs, Achilles tendonitis, tennis elbow, and shoulder tendonitis.

I discovered the benefits of a low-tech approach myself after fracturing my shoulder while running a few years ago. My arm was still in excruciating pain when I visited my orthopedist for a follow-up. I asked if I'd need an operation.

"Probably not," he replied, eyeing my x-rays distractedly. I thought I detect-ed disappointment in his voice. "We'll see if it heals right first."

"Is there anything I can do to help it?" I asked.

He made a little gesture with his arm and said, "Just rotate it like this." Then he grabbed my chart and made his getaway.

Dissatisfied, I consulted another orthopedist who went the extra mile to show me which exercises would speed my recovery—even though it meant she wouldn't be performing more lucrative surgery.

The nice thing was that she empowered me to affect my outcome. I dutifully performed the exercises, happy in the knowledge that each painful stretch was reducing my chances of chronic aching and stiffness. And sure enough, though it took nearly a year, my arm recovered without surgery. Today, I can bench-press more than my own bodyweight, pain free. The shoulder is literally better than ever.

Diversify Your Athletic Portfolio

Bottom-line: Boomers need to be less fixated on athletic perfection. I see examples of this everyday with my patients. There's the fifty-eight-year-old guy who wants to keep running marathons but has knee pain from calcifications. He typically runs thirty to forty miles a week, yet when he can't get out because of pain or injury, he grows despondent, consoles himself with sugary snacks and gains weight.

Then there's the sixty-five-year-old "gray fox," still super-fit in his tennis togs. He's disappointed with the "crick" in his shoulder that has slowed his overhead serves. Even though his orthopedist is reluctant to operate, my patient's desire for a performance-enhancing quick-fix may soon land him in the arthroscopy suite.

I might have become one of these single-minded zealots myself, if not for the back pain that began when I was in medical school. Back then I focused almost exclusively on long-distance running, religiously pounding the pavement of Manhattan to push my endurance. Not only had I placed all my exercise eggs in one basket, but also I wasn't dealing effectively with stress. The dividends eventually stopped paying out; my back pain got worse and running got harder.

I might have delivered myself to a back specialist where an MRI would likely have revealed compressed discs in my back (they invariably do!). And chances are I'd have received a series of injections and high-tech operations to get me sprinting again.

Instead, I took the advice of a friend—an inveterate bicyclist who'd started kayaking after being sidelined by knee pain—and resolved to *diversify my exercise portfolio.* I took up kayaking, too, and also started strength training. I added ten pounds of healthy muscle to my gaunt runner's frame. I also retired from marathons and instead took up triathlons, which distribute training stress among three different aerobic disciplines: running, swimming, and bicycling. In addition, I became more alert to psychological tensions that put "voltage" into my back circuits.

Since then, I've had virtually complete relief from back pain. I no longer cringe at the prospect of moving furniture or loading a car or even bending to tie my shoes. If I get an occasional twinge of pain, it doesn't mean weeks of aching and immobilization. I simply adjust my exercise routine and things get better. I'm no champion, but I'm still in the game, while other boomers have succumbed to their own obsessive zeal.

HEADING OFF ARTHRITIC CONDITIONS

With more than one hundred types of arthritis, it's often hard to get a handle on what exactly the disease is. One thing every type shares is pain, stiffness, and joint swelling that make it hard to move around and engage in daily tasks.

Two of the most common forms are rheumatoid arthritis (where the immune system attacks the tissues lining the joints) and osteoarthritis (the "wear-and-tear" breakdown of cartilage that causes bones to rub together painfully at the joints). Though they're different, many of the prevention and treatment strategies discussed in this chapter apply to both, as well as many other kinds of arthritis.

A Holistic Approach + Patience

Because my mother's rheumatoid arthritis (RA) began in her forties, I never took joint health for granted. I was fine until I hit my early forties and noticed something strange: my curiously double-jointed thumbs—long a party curiosity and conversation-starter—began to ache. When the first one started throbbing, I assumed I'd just strained it. But when both became stiff and painful simultaneously, I couldn't avoid the truth: *I* was in the beginning stages of middle-age arthritis.

I ran the usual blood tests, but found nothing amiss. Obviously, I was auditioning for a full-blown case of RA (likely inherited from my mother), but had not yet landed the role. But what to do about it?

In the "old days" when I was in training, RA was thought to be an incurable disease. Pain killers could relieve its discomforts, and if it got too serious or threatened to cause irreversible deformity, then patients were urged to try drugs called DMARDs (disease-modifying anti-rheumatic drugs). DMARDs, like prednisone, gold shots, methotrexate (a chemotherapy drug), and Plaquenil (an anti-parasite drug), were moderately effective, but could cause dangerous side effects. Extreme solutions—even whole-body radiation to suppress the immune system from attacking joint tissues—were tried and abandoned after serious consequences outweighed potential benefits.

The biotech revolution yielded yet another new crop of drugs—monoclonal antibodies. These drugs were carefully designed to sweep away molecules that trigger inflammation—specifically tumor necrosis factor alpha (TNF). However, it doesn't take a rocket scientist to figure out that eliminating something that suppresses tumors might result in cancer *promotion*. And, indeed, that's precisely what happened. Lymphoma rates are several times higher in those who take these costly drugs. And because the immune system is blunted, their susceptibility to infections is greater, including dermatological problems, like skin ulcers and eczema.

The advent of monoclonal antibody drugs, like Enbrel, Humira, and Remicade, also radically changed the RA treatment philosophy. Suddenly, physicians were urged to drop the dime on RA early—*before* serious irreversible joint damage occurred. While this might be reasonable in some cases, market pressure is now on to sign patients up for very expensive and possibly hazardous drug regimens without trying more conservative treatments first. Unfortunately, this makes it tougher for holistic doctors like me to grab a window of opportunity for our approaches—many of which are surprisingly effective, but take longer to work. Instant gratification it's *not*.

Crisis of Faith

I learned this myself the hard way after opting for an aggressive nutritional program instead of conventional treatments to relieve my aching thumbs. I religiously took fish oil, antioxidants, glucosamine and chondroitin, MSM, and natural anti-inflammatories, like curcumin, EGCG from green tea, and boswellin (all are discussed later in this chapter). I also strictly adhered to my own Salad and Salmon Diet, further eliminating wheat and dairy after testing allergic to both.

After six weeks, though, I still hadn't seen any improvement! I began to doubt my approach—and even briefly considered opening up some Celebrex samples left by a drug rep before thinking better of it. And then I had a revelation: instead

WHICH NATURAL INTERVENTIONS WORK BEST?		
Intervention	**Rheumatoid Arthritis**	**Osteoarthritis**
Boswellin	Prevent, treat	Prevent, treat
Cat's Claw	Treat	Research inconclusive
Diet	Prevent, treat	Prevent, treat
Exercise	Treat	Prevent, treat
Fish Oil	Prevent, treat	Prevent, treat
Glucosamine/Chondroitin	Research inconclusive	Prevent, treat
MSM	Prevent, treat	Prevent, treat
Natural Cox-2 Inhibitors	Treat	Treat
UC-II	Treat	Research inconclusive
Vitamin D	Prevent, treat	Research inconclusive

of caving into the pain, I had to practice what I preached and hang on for another few weeks until these slower-acting natural methods could work their relief.

And therein lies the rub—natural arthritis treatments take time, patience and, yes, a certain amount of *faith* to see results. While patients may note some improvements in just a few weeks, the ultimate benefits of diet modification, supplementation, and proper exercise often aren't evident for twelve to eighteen months. And their full potential may not be realized for *two to three years*! For an RA sufferer with rampaging symptoms, this may not be fast enough. In these cases, I have patients team their conventional medications with natural interventions, checking frequently to see that they're responding well.

In my own case, faith was rewarded. Gradually, my symptoms got better, and after a year I regained my role as thumb-popping "life of the party." To this day, I remain arthritis free and credit this to steadfast adherence to my maintenance program.

TELL YOUR DOCTOR ABOUT THESE

If you suspect you're developing arthritis or already have it, you may want to try some or all of the following evidence-based CAM therapies. Discuss them with your doctor first. The chart "Which Natural Interventions Work Best" on page 138 provides an easy reference. See Resources for Patients for more on these treatments.

Boswellin

Derived from gum resin from the bark of the *Boswellia serrata* tree, this anti-inflammatory has been used for centuries by Ayurvedic healers to relieve arthritic conditions. For osteoarthritis and RA symptoms, try one 150-mg supplement three times a day.

Cat's Claw

This rainforest herb has long been used as a traditional remedy for arthritic problems in South America. It's now taking its place in modern medicine alongside such established Amazon remedies as quinine for malaria and curare for surgical anesthesia.

Recent research confirms cat's claw's potential against RA. Not only is it a powerful natural antioxidant, but test tube studies show it also imitates the inflammation-quenching activity of powerful monoclonal antibody drugs.[4] Early research also suggests it may prevent NSAID-induced gastric irritation. For arthritis symptoms, I recommend one capsule (250 mg) twice daily. One caveat: If you're already taking one of the monoclonal antibody drugs, you may want to forgo the potentially unwelcome additive effects of cat's claw.

Fish Oil

My colleague, William Campbell Douglas III, M.D., recalls being chastised during his residency in 1989 for putting one of his arthritis patients on fish oil. The residency director ordered him to stick to the "standard of care." When he argued that there was no such thing since medicine is a constantly changing art and science, things got heated. He almost quit after his internship but ultimately decided not to be cowed by such "standards of scare."

Evidence has since proven him right. Omega-3 fatty acids in fish oil appear to work similarly to monoclonal antibody drugs by gently suppressing pro-inflammatory molecules like TNF alpha. Only fish oil works more slowly, and there's no evidence that its gentle immune suppression raises the risk of infections or cancer—in fact, as we saw in the last chapter fish oil is linked with lowered risk of many cancers.

To prevent arthritis take two 1,000-milligram (mg) fish-oil capsules per day containing 420 mg of the fatty acid EPA (eicosapentaenoic acid) and 300 mg of DHA (docosahexaenoic acid). For treatment, take six to nine capsules per day. See Chapter 6 for more on the best fish sources and supplements.

There's also another part to the story: refined vegetable oils and hydrogenated fats in junk foods may have the exact opposite effect of omega-3s. In other words, they may promote inflammation by acting as precursors to a powerful pro-inflammatory agent—arachidonic acid. Unfortunately, today's diets—bereft of omega-3s and rich in omega-6s and synthetic fats—have resulted in an imbalance of essential fatty acids (EFAs) and even more inflammation. The ideal ratio is about 1 (omega-6):1 (omega-3). However, most Americans average from 20:1 to 50:1. This can actually be detected via an EFA blood profile (see Chapter 4).

I tell my patients that by reducing their intake of harmful omega-6s and boosting their intake of omega-3s (that means fewer processed crackers, packaged snacks, and french fries and more cold-water fish, nuts, and flaxseeds) they can have a significant impact on their arthritis.

Glucosamine/Chondroitin

These two natural substances, which aid in repairing and maintaining cartilage health, are practically poster children for the proposition of this book—that cutting-edge natural therapies can, after extensive research and clinical experience, make their way to the forefront of conventional medical practice. Today, most rheumatologists and orthopedists encourage their patients with mild complaints to give glucosamine and chondroitin a try. But this wasn't always the case.

I first became aware of glucosamine via a horse-fanciers magazine. I'd gotten into riding and somehow was placed on a mailing list for equestrians. Amid ads

for riding jodhpurs and saddles, I saw a full-page spread for "Cosequin," a glucosamine formula that came in a bucket. When added to horse feed, it healed strained
fetlocks (a joint above the hoof). Soon afterward, glucosamine for humans hit the
market.

Jason Theodosakis, M.D., author of *The Arthritis Cure,* has long been a proponent of glucosamine and chondroitin for osteoarthritis (it may also offer relief
for RA) and favors teaming them with ASU (avocado and soy unsaponifiables).
Research in France has shown this substance—marketed overseas as Piascledine—
to be remarkably effective against arthritis. Dr. Theodosakis offers his own brand,
called Avosoy (see Resources for Patients).

Lactoferrin

Because many people combine CAM therapies with conventional therapies, like
NSAIDs, they may still be vulnerable to the bleeding side effects of these powerful drugs. New research now suggests that lactoferrin (a natural iron-binding milk
protein), taken in supplement form, can help curb NSAID-related problems like
ulcers and intestinal bleeding.[5] Lactoferrin has antibiotic and anti-inflammatory
properties that repair the intestine by sequestering iron (a free-radical promoter)
and protect the gastrointestinal tract from NSAID damage. If you're taking
NSAIDs, try one to three lactoferrin capsules at night before bed or as directed
by a doctor.

Natural Cox-2 Inhibitors

Several herbs exhibit natural anti-inflammatory properties, similar to popular
COX-2 inhibitors. In truth, these natural wanna-bes are neither as rapid acting
nor as devastating in their side effects as their pharmaceutical counterparts. But
their gentle, gradual anti-inflammatory actions make them safe, worthwhile
accompaniments to fish oil and other natural arthritis therapies.

  • **Curcumin:** One of the most potent anti-inflammatories, curcumin is an
  extract of the culinary herb turmeric, used in curry. For arthritis relief, try one
  capsule twice daily with food.

  • **Green tea:** Another potent natural anti-inflammatory is green tea. But to
  obtain its benefits, you'd need to drink at least fifteen to twenty cups a day. I
  therefore have developed an ultra-potent encapsulated green tea extract called
  EGCG Ultra, containing 500 mg of 70 percent EGCG per capsule (the equivalent of fifteen to twenty cups of green tea). For arthritis relief, take one capsule with food twice daily. For those who want the combined benefits of
  curcumin and green tea, as well as other anti-inflammatory herbs like rosemary,
  basil, oregano, and ginger, try one to two capsules of Zyflamend twice daily.

- **Bromelain:** This extract from pineapple stems is an example of another broad category of natural products used to treat inflammatory conditions: enzymes. Bromelain is used extensively in Europe and the United States as a complementary therapy in rheumatology and sports medicine. Take 200–2,000 mg per day in four doses, with or without food. A popular supplement that combines the anti-inflammatory effects of bromelain with other important enzymes is Wobenzym. Take one to three tablets four times daily for arthritis or injuries.

MSM

This natural form of organic sulfur (methylsulfonylmethane) gained clout in 1999 after actor James Coburn won the Oscar for Best Supporting Actor and credited it with helping him overcome RA. Sulfur is a natural constituent of cartilage that

THE LOW-DOWN ON DRUG/NUTRIENT INTERACTIONS

Recently I ran across this lurid headline on the popular Reuters Health website: "Herbal Remedies Put Arthritis Patients at Risk of Harmful Interactions." Not only is this a case study in unwarranted conclusions, but it also does a profound disservice to patients and doctors.

- **Risky herbal remedies:** Based on new research, the news story reported on *theoretical,* not actual drug interactions. Indeed, the study's only real finding was the vague assertion that 44 percent of patients at a British orthopedic clinic took herbal or OTC remedies in the previous six months.[6] From this it inferred that 11 percent of them were taking remedies like garlic, echinacea, ginger, devil's claw, or ginkgo biloba that put them at risk for serious interactions with conventional arthritis drugs, such as NSAIDs and DMARDs. However, at no time during the study did any patient actually experience adverse side effects from these "risky" combinations.

  A comprehensive search of Applied Nutrition's Drug-Nutrient Workshop database (www.nutritionworkshop.com) revealed no known or even theoretical reactions between the drugs in question and the supplements. The only exception was echinacea, which can reduce blood levels of certain medications, but hasn't been documented to cause harm. Even so, the ominous and unwarranted conclusion was that patients are harming themselves in droves.

- **Balancing the evidence:** The theoretical risk of arthritis drug/supplement combos is exaggerated, in my opinion. Nevertheless, I always caution patients may be deficient in arthritic joints. MSM appears to deliver needed sulfur, offering pain relief and reducing inflammation.

For arthritis, take a 1,000 mg capsule twice daily, working up slowly to one-half teaspoon of powdered MSM (2,500 mg) twice daily. Try it in green tea to hide the bitter taste. Note: High doses may sometimes cause diarrhea.

Stress Reduction

Your pain might just be in your brain after all. A recent study of children with arthritis shows that higher stress and moodiness correlates to a rise in arthritis symptoms, including pain, fatigue, and stiffness.[7]

The study confirms what researchers have long suspected: non-drug therapies, such as stress management, relaxation techniques, and cognitive behavioral

against combining powerful conventional drugs with poorly labeled or minimally identified herbal concoctions (see "Too Good to Be True" on page 148 for tips on discussing "hyped" but unproven therapies with your doctor). For example, I once had a celebrity patient who swore by the joint relief he got from "Chinese black balls," purchased in Hong Kong. I urged caution after I inspected the crudely manufactured spheres, which came in little cellophane bags with no directions or ingredient list. It wasn't until later that the story broke about bootleg Chinese herbal pills for arthritis—laced with dangerous levels of powerful NSAIDs, steroids, and Valium.

I also discourage the use of white willow bark, the herbal precursor to modern aspirin, in combination with other anti-inflammatories. On its own, it causes minimal gastric irritation and bleeding, but used with other drugs, the risk is heightened.

That's not to say, though, that certain natural arthritis therapies aren't excellent complements to conventional remedies. For instance, arthritis sufferers who combine fish oil and glucosamine with NSAIDs tend to have more pain-free days, allowing them to step down use of conventional medications. Plus, fish oil counteracts the drawbacks of NSAIDs (gastrointestinal bleeding, blood pressure spikes, and cardiac problems) by healing gastric tissue, lowering blood pressure, and improving heart function.

• **Bottom-line:** Arthritis sufferers who judiciously combine their medications with supplements—under the supervision of knowledgeable health professionals—often obtain considerable synergistic benefits.

therapy, have significant potential to relieve arthritis symptoms. Ask your doctor for a referral to someone with expertise in stress reduction.

Undenatured Collagen Type II

A few years ago, I learned of interesting research on a form of chicken collagen, undenatured collagen type II (UC II, for short), that seemed to ameliorate rheumatoid arthritis.[8] Imagine how surprised I was to find that the concept originated in the laboratories of David E. Trentham, M.D., an acknowledged leader in *conventional* arthritis research at Harvard.

I later met Dr. Trentham at an arthritis conference. He provided an excellent review of drug therapies for arthritis, but made no mention of UC II. After the lecture, I introduced myself and asked him about it. Looking around as if embarrassed, he allowed that research was proceeding.

Later, I saw him lecture enthusiastically about UC II at several complementary medicine conferences, as if he'd finally come out of the closet. I say this not to disparage Dr. Trentham, but to illustrate the barricades distinguished researchers often encounter as they embrace more "out of the box" therapies.

UC II works via the process of "oral tolerization"—reducing symptoms by introducing minute amounts of the very substance (in this case, collagen) targeted by the autoimmune system. It's as if the chicken collagen "runs interference" for an over-exuberant immune system. UC II seems to work best against RA, but since osteoarthritis shares certain autoimmune characteristics with RA, I've also found it helpful for OA patients.

Take 5–10 mg of UC II at bedtime.

Vitamin D

African Americans with RA report more debilitating symptoms and severe disability than whites. Experts have attributed this disparity to any number of factors: genes, poverty-related poor diet, and even the effects of racial differences in care. Now there's an intriguing new theory: vitamin D deficiency.

In fact, dark-skinned people seem uniquely predisposed to this deficiency, which is now clearly linked to autoimmune diseases like multiple sclerosis and RA. The reason is this: dark skin is a protective adaptation to equatorial sunlight, slowing down absorption of ultraviolet B rays (which trigger vitamin D production in the body) to just the right amount—as long as the sun shines constantly. In less sunny northern climates, however, dark skin's additional defenses against already scarce ultraviolet B rays can quickly result in D deficiency.

My point isn't to single out African Americans; I use this example merely to illustrate a possible link between RA and vitamin D deficiency. Interestingly, vitamin D deficiency is also increasingly common in light-skinned whites now that they're urged to stay out of the sun or slather on sunscreen. My real message is that supplementing with vitamin D may be a key component of any arthritis-prevention plan.

Even if you don't suffer from arthritis, but merely have "aching bones," you may benefit from D supplementation, according to Dr. Michael Holick, a leading vitamin D researcher. Holick and other researchers have discovered that those with low vitamin D levels may suffer from osteomalacia (softening of the bones), which leads to vague aching. For more on vitamin D and sun exposure, read Dr. Holick's book *The UV Advantage.*

TIP: If you suffer from arthritis or aching, have your doctor measure your vitamin D levels (see Chapter 4). If they're low, take 1,000–4,000 international units (IU) of natural vitamin D3, while monitoring D levels frequently until it's in the high-normal range. Or get controlled exposure to sunlight (fifteen to forty-five minutes per day, depending on your level of skin pigment). In northern latitudes this is only effective from April to October.

REVISITING CONTROVERSIES

The following arthritis prevention and treatment strategies—though more controversial than those listed above—are nonetheless worth discussing with your doctor.

Mediterranean Diet and Arthritis

Early in my career, the Arthritis Foundation was an implacable foe of "diet quackery." Thankfully, with new advances in science and the recognition that patients are clamoring for lifestyle answers to lessen the effects of powerful drugs, this has changed. Consult the Foundation's website and you'll read the following:

> There are scientific reasons to think that the foods you eat could affect certain kinds of arthritis. Evidence shows that excessive weight and the type of diet you follow may influence symptoms of certain types of arthritis and related conditions.[9]

Though cautiously conservative, the Foundation now acknowledges that diet *can* play a role in osteoarthritis, RA, and other arthritic diseases. At the very least, it allows that weight loss reduces wear and tear on joints.

But obesity's deleterious effects are more than just a gravity problem. Overweight also creates a metabolic propensity to inflammation, which has a role in arthritis, just as it does in heart disease and cancer. Patients have long noted that various diets are therapeutic against joint pain. Unfortunately, many conventional doctors either don't know much about diet or don't believe it can help.

Perhaps the most decisive confirmation of the diet-arthritis connection comes from Swedish research showing that fasting results in a striking reduction in rheu-matoid arthritis symptoms and progression.[10] Not exactly a practical solution, but it nevertheless makes a point!

Since then, studies have noted that the Mediterranean diet, comprised of tra-ditional foods from Crete (think fresh fruits, vegetables, whole breads/grains, beans, nuts, seeds, olive oil, and fish) can also slow disease activity.[11] Most likely, it's the absence of refined foods, the preponderance of dietary polyphenols from plant sources, and the anti–inflammatory effects of abundant omega–3-rich fish that make the difference. Even if your doctor doesn't push you to change your diet, consider doing so yourself. Like the Mediterranean diet, my Salad and Salmon Diet is also helpful in preventing and treating all types of arthritis. See Chapter 6 or visit my website at www.drhoffman.com/page.cfm/21. (Also see "Gout Diet" below.)

GOUT DIET

When the body is unable to properly eliminate uric acid, the result can be a type of arthritis called gout. Too much uric acid (formed from the breakdown of dietary purines) causes painful needlelike crystals to form in the joints.

Purines are actually *ribonucleic acids* that carry the code for protein synthesis in cells. So they're found abundantly in the cells of certain high-protein foods, such as meats, seeds, beans, and certain vegetables, like asparagus and spinach. They're also found in whole grains, which retain the protein-rich material from seed germs (the reproductive area where the seed germinates to form a sprout). For this rea-son, individuals with gout are encouraged to eat low-purine foods, such as refined flours (without seed germs) and protein foods that don't contain cells, like dairy products and eggs. (A list of low-purine foods can be found at www.healthsquare.com/mc/fgmc2005.htm.)

But there's more to gout than purines. By loading up on "permissible" foods, like white bread, white rice, refined pasta, fruits, juices, and low-fat dairy prod-ucts, gout sufferers can inadvertently set themselves up for insulin resistance (see Chapter 6). Therefore, I like to recommend certain features of the Salad and Salmon diet for gout patients with a few modifications. Like other gout diets, I urge curb-ing high-purine meats, beans, and vegetables, while substituting more eggs and dairy. But instead of low-purine refined carbohydrates, I recommend more low-glycemic foods (slower-acting carbohydrates, such as whole grains, that don't raise blood sugar quickly and elevate insulin production). See www.glycemicindex.com for more information.

Exercise and Arthritis

Time was when arthritis sufferers were cautioned not to exercise for fear it would damage already inflamed, painful joints. Not only has research ruled this out, but also one new study even suggests that regular *vigorous* exercise is better yet.[12]

Researchers followed more than 5,700 older adults with arthritis for two years. Those who didn't exercise vigorously at least three times a week—such as doing heavy housework or playing a sport—doubled their risk of physical decline. This included not being able to carry out basic everyday activities, like bathing, cooking, and shopping.

Your doctor may not say much about the benefits of exercise for arthritis—and certainly won't urge you to scale Mount Everest or take up snowboarding. But you might consider non-joint-punishing workouts in the pool (swimming, water aerobics, and aqua jogging). See Resources for Patients for more on arthritis exercises.

Additionally, new equipment options, like the elliptical trainer and recumbent bicycle have made for kinder, gentler aerobic workouts. Elliptical trainers are similar to treadmills but have pedals, offering a smoother, no-impact workout. Recumbent bikes are equipped with a backrest for support.

Don't be scared of weight training either. Universal equipment is designed to minimize range-of-motion mistakes that damage joints. But start slowly with twelve to fifteen repetitions at moderate intensity, rather than the six to eight at full tilt (favored by bodybuilders). Also, be sure to get some equipment-safety advice from a certified professional trainer or physical therapist.

Unfortunately, many arthritis sufferers experience such severe joint pain that strenuous exercise is out of the question. For them, yoga provides an excellent alternative. Preliminary research at the University of Pennsylvania on individuals with severe osteoarthritis of the knee suggests that even a short eight-week program of yoga can yield significant improvements in their ability to walk and lessen pain dramatically.[13]

Avoid heavy yoga workouts, like yogaerobics—a prime example of a gentle tradition that's been "lost in translation." For yoga to be effective, try it at least three to four times a week, either in a class or at home. Check your local "Y" or hospital for classes near you.

Tip: Some arthritis sufferers report better results with Bikram yoga—a rigorous form performed in a room heated to at least 95°F.

Magnet Therapy

Once synonymous with arthritis quackery, scientific evidence is reviving this ancient self-treatment for pain. But not all doctors are convinced that it works.

The idea behind magnets is that they help restore the normal electromagnetic balance thrown off by injury or inflammation. Applying them to painful areas appears to improve blood flow, allowing in more healing nutrients and oxygen.

In a recent study at McMasters University in Ontario, 194 men and women with arthritis of the hip and knee were fitted with magnetic bracelets or dummy placebo bracelets.[14] Researchers found that the magnets offered a slight but real effect on pain and mobility, confirming the results of several previous studies.

Magnet therapy is non-invasive and safe, but effectiveness depends on the strength of the magnet and length of time it's applied (see Resources for Patients for reliable sources). Magnets can be applied daily or at night while sleeping, but avoid applying them close to the brain or visceral organs where they may interfere with the body's normal electrical impulses. They're also not recommended during pregnancy.

TOO GOOD TO BE TRUE

Not every CAM therapy is ready for prime time, but many are slickly marketed as "sure things" to unsuspecting patients. Unfortunately, when doctors try to set patients straight, conflicts often arise. With mutual respect and patience, though, this needn't be the case.

Sally Theis, a sixty-five-year-old arthritis sufferer, recently received a flyer in the mail touting a "Remarkable New Arthritis Breakthrough." The pitch was for a "powerful natural anti-inflammatory" herb found only in the jungles of New Guinea, where anthropologists report that people are "free of arthritis and other degenerative diseases."*

Excited by these seeming scientific claims and the possibility of finding real relief for her painful arthritis, Sally made an appointment with her doctor to talk about trying the herb for herself. However, her doctor wasn't impressed—and for good reason. Here, they sort through the hype and eventually reach a compromise.

Dr. Carson: Sally, I agree this *sounds* promising, but we all need to be careful with buzzwords, like "breakthrough" and "cure." I hate to say it, but a lot of companies send targeted mailings—typically to older people like you who live in affluent areas and frequently buy health products.

Sally: It's just that this one sounds better than most. It actually has a bibliography listing journal articles and has lots of detailed drawings and scientific explanations.

Acupuncture

Another frequently maligned ancient remedy is acupuncture. Your doctor may discount its ability to relieve arthritis pain because acupuncture has often proven difficult to test. Part of the problem is that the mere act of sticking in needles and receiving attention can generate a substantial placebo response. That is, patients may get relief from arthritis pain either because they believe acupuncture will work or because they are responding positively to some other aspect of the therapeutic experience.

Researchers have now solved this conundrum by comparing real acupuncture to "sham" acupuncture where needles are stuck into random, non-responsive sites rather than true acupuncture points. In the largest study of its kind, involving 570 patients with knee osteoarthritis, acupuncture was finally vindicated.[15] After a series of twenty-five treatments over six months, patients in the true

Dr. Carson: I know you're willing to try almost anything to stop the pain. Believe me, I'd love to give you a clear go-ahead on this. But let's look at some of these research citations. Most are from obscure journals and refer to test tube experiments that show how the herb acts on inflammation in isolated cartilage cells. The key is there are *no* human studies yet.

Sally: How do you explain why tribal people who use it don't have arthritis?

Dr. Carson: It could be their natural diet or a lifetime of exercise or the fact that most die young from snakebites and wild boar attacks before they're old enough to get arthritis. We simply don't know because it hasn't been studied. Here's what I suggest. Let's both take a look at the American Botanical Council's *HerbalGram* database (www.herbalgram.org). It's good for sorting through emerging therapies. Then let's talk again.

After more research, they both agree that little is really known about the herb, either negative or positive. Dr. Carson cautions that the best approach is to wait until more reliable information emerges. However, he reluctantly agrees that Sally can try it as long as she allows him to monitor her. See Chapter 3 for more on interpreting medical research.

* The herb and medical claims are hypothetical.

acupuncture group experienced significant improvement in pain and function compared with the sham acupuncture group.

Unfortunately, finding a qualified acupuncturist isn't always easy. The National Certification Commission for Acupuncture and Oriental Medicine (NCCAOM) has an online directory of board-certified practitioners (www.nccaom.org/home. htm). Many states also license acupuncturists. But some of the most gifted practitioners practice off the beaten path, as did some of my uncertified teachers who were superbly trained in their Asian countries of origin. Likewise, some Western-trained acupuncturists, even medical doctors, have achieved academic proficiency, but lack the superb needle skills of their more experienced, less-credentialed Asian-trained colleagues. In other words, proceed with an open mind and follow your instincts.

Gluten Connection

Looked at narrowly, celiac disease is strictly an ailment of the gastrointestinal tract caused by intolerance to gluten (a component of wheat, barley, rye, and other grains). But in my experience, gluten sensitivity may also be an underlying contributor to various forms of arthritis. This makes sense—though not to many conventional doctors—because gluten pushes the immune system into overdrive in susceptible individuals, resulting in inflammation and tissue destruction throughout the body. When the target is the joints, arthritis arises.

Research is beginning to confirm my controversial proposition. A recent study describes three patients with lupus whose symptoms were substantially improved when they eliminated gluten from their diets after doctors discovered anti-gliadin antibodies (indicating possible gluten sensitivity).[16] If you suspect celiac disease, ask your doctor to test you (see Chapter 4).

Natural Hormone Replacement

Some complementary physicians, like me, have adopted a new but controversial approach to inflammatory disorders: the use of natural androgenic, or male, hormones to "quench" the inflammatory cascade.

Research has demonstrated that DHEA, an androgenic precursor to both testosterone and estrogen, can dramatically reduce lupus symptoms in women. Lupus is an autoimmune disease, which attacks healthy tissue, causing it to become swollen and painful. One common target is joints, resulting in a type of arthritis.

Like DHEA, testosterone also appears to keep inflammation at bay.[17] In fact, RA has been linked to both low testosterone and low DHEA levels. What's more, prednisone, a synthetic steroid frequently given for serious inflammatory arthritis, tends to suppress the body's production of testosterone and DHEA. For this reason, I recommend testing hormone levels in men (and women) with inflammatory rheumatoid conditions and normalizing their testosterone and DHEA under a doctor's supervision (see Chapter 4). Practitioners familiar with prescribing natural hormones may be found on the American College for Advancement in Medicine's website (www.acam.org).

Despite the prevalence of arthritic diseases, medical researchers still don't fully understand the mechanics behind their development and progression. Indeed, as we've seen, there may be multiple factors at play, including a nutrition connection, a hormonal connection, a stress connection, and even an allergy connection.

A holistic approach to preventing and managing arthritis and orthopedic problems includes paying attention to all these components and fashioning an individualized treatment plan (emphasizing gentler natural therapies) that addresses underlying problems.

In the next chapter, we'll explore how a similar approach can be used to prevent or minimize cognitive declines and memory problems.

Cognitive Problems

Feeeed your head . . .

—GRACE SLICK, JEFFERSON AIRPLANE

A strange transition has occurred as the baby boom generation approaches Social Security age. Millions of boomers who spent the 1960s and 1970s experimenting with mind-altering substances to achieve the kind of insight promised by then-popular authors like Herman Hesse (*Siddhartha*) and Ken Kesey (*One Flew Over the Cuckoo's Nest*) are now obsessed with optimizing (not deconstructing) their mental performance. They place a high premium on preserving their memory and avoiding the cognitive declines that often accompany aging.

Patients in their forties, fifties, and sixties constantly visit me, concerned that their cognitive capabilities are dwindling, and demanding innovative solutions. Some have a parent recently diagnosed with Alzheimer's disease. Others are women embarking on a second career after raising a family who find their mental skills suddenly rusty. Many are simply aging members of the increasingly digital workforce, worried about being left behind in the race for productivity.

Of course, some of their concerns are real. Studies show that memory and mental performance decline at a predictable, steady rate after age forty. In fact, as many as one in five people over seventy who don't have dementia may nevertheless have mild cognitive impairment (low-level memory loss that can increase risk for Alzheimer's disease).

Looked at another way, though, that means a majority of older people don't have any cognitive impairment at all. Indeed, recent research shows that many people approaching the century mark exhibit absolutely no sign of memory loss or cognitive decline, and just one-third have actual dementia (a catch-all phrase for several debilitating cognitive diseases, including Alzheimer's disease).[1] In other words, mental declines may be linked to aging, but aren't inevitable. What's more, older people might actually be better than younger people at discerning "the big picture," even if they occasionally forget the everyday details of life. This used to be called wisdom, and before the advent of today's throwaway, youth-oriented culture, the "tribal elder" was prized.

In this chapter we'll look at natural ways to lessen the impact of aging on cognition and boost brain power at any age. As with previous chapters, we'll also explore natural therapies that may halt or even reverse certain types of cognitive decline. Plus, we'll revisit some controversial treatments that may well be worth discussing with your doctor.

DO I HAVE ALZHEIMER'S DISEASE?

Sally was a typical, worried-well boomer of forty-eight. Her father had recently been diagnosed with Alzheimer's disease, which was troubling enough. But her new duties as caregiver had added considerably to her apprehension and stress. With her kids in college, Sally was also completing her Master's in Social Work and hoped for a new career as a psychotherapist. But she was having trouble focusing on her heavy workload and competing against twenty-somethings. A conscientious straight-A student in college, her confidence was shattered when she got Bs on her midterms.

After examining Sally, I reassured her that the problems she was experiencing sounded fairly typical and didn't arouse my suspicion for Alzheimer's disease. She appreciated the reality check, but was still concerned.

After talking further, several key themes emerged: 1) Sally was a tense, stressed-out perfectionist, and her current life situation wasn't conducive to optimal cognitive performance; 2) Sally was in the throes of menopause, rendering her "brain-dead" due to hormonal factors; 3) Sally was at the mercy of fluxes in blood sugar, which were further impairing her cognitive function. On the following pages, we'll see how addressing these themes and others can minimize and even stop cognitive decline.

Nature or Nurture?

Like cancer researchers, cognitive scientists are discovering that serious age-related mental deterioration, including Alzheimer's disease and even mild cognitive impairment, can often be predicted early. The hope is to eventually find effective treatments to head them off before nerve cell deterioration and major memory loss renders patients unable to function in everyday life.

Early results are promising. Studies now show that tests measuring recall and learning in older people are effective at predicting who will go on to develop mild cognitive impairment and even Alzheimer's disease. Those with increased memory slips over time are most at risk. Brain scans also show early promise for detecting Alzheimer's, sometimes years before symptoms show up.

In addition, geneticists are exploring whether some people carry Alzheimer's disease or dementia genes (though the hereditary connection remains murky). Consider these facts:

• No single gene is responsible for all cases of Alzheimer's disease. In fact, the vast majority of Alzheimer's cases aren't the result of an inherited genetic defect at all. Even having one or two close relatives (parents or siblings) with the disease doesn't necessarily mean the cause is genetic if you get it.

• Only about 50 percent of people with a strong family history of early-onset Alzheimer's disease (which is linked to a few specific genetic defects and usually manifests before the age of sixty-five), appear to inherit a faulty gene. However, almost all people who do inherit one go on to develop early Alzheimer's disease.

• Some cases of late-onset Alzheimer's disease (in people sixty-five and older) also have a genetic component linked to a gene called apolipoprotein E (ApoE). However, the connection is much weaker than in early-onset Alzheimer's. Carrying one of the three ApoE genes boosts your chances of getting the disease to varying degrees, but doesn't guarantee it. Obviously, additional factors are at play.

• Other forms of dementia can also be inherited, though they're rare. Like Alzheimer's disease, the majority of dementias appear to develop via a combination of factors.

Deciding Whether to Test

Like Sally, most baby boomers have high expectations. Not only do they expect their bodies to continue plugging away at sixty like they did at twenty, but they also count on their minds to remain razor-sharp well into old age. Rather than gracefully accepting that car keys are occasionally misplaced and appointments forgotten, many middle-aged boomers assume these "senior moments" mean they're well on the way to full-fledged dementia. This is particularly true if they've watched a parent gradually slip out of cognitive reach. The inevitable thought: "What if it's genetic?"

The decision to get tested for an Alzheimer's gene is personal. If you have two or more close family members who developed the disease before age sixty-five (early-onset Alzheimer's disease), you might benefit most from genetic counseling and testing. For one thing, knowing early that you carry a gene allows you to take advantage of early interventions (including the natural brain boosters discussed in this chapter).

However, because sure-fire treatments aren't yet available to fix genetic defects, there's no guarantee that any interventions will stave off disease. Genetic testing may simply sentence you to perpetual anxiety because not every Alzheimer's gene means certain disease nor does every negative test ensure you're off the hook. Always talk to your doctor or a genetic counselor about the pros and cons before deciding to test.

Other Memory Blockers

Many memory blips are temporary and may be linked to environmental or emotional factors rather than to disease. In other words, don't assume the worst or let medical jargon scare you into a condition you don't have (see "Say What? Making Sense of Doctorese" below). Your forgetfulness and cloudy thinking might just be the fog of stress, depression, anxiety, or even pessimism. All are linked to temporary memory loss. However, if allowed to continue, these emotional states can actually raise your risk of dementia (particularly pessimism).

SAY WHAT? MAKING SENSE OF DOCTORESE

Your doctor probably believes she's speaking plain English. But it could be Singhalese, for all you know. Medical jargon is at best indecipherable, and at worst, downright frightening . . . particularly when it comes to cognitive problems. Consider this perplexing information one patient received after her brain MRI came back negative (clear): "Very tiny area of increased signal in the left centrum semiovale nonspecific. This is a non-enhancing area and is nonspecific."

Huh? What the doctor meant to say is that a small quantity of contrast fluid (injected into the bloodstream to enhance resolution in the scanned area) is leaking into the brain tissue. "Non-specific" means there's no apparent disease causing the leak. In other words, it should be watched but probably isn't anything to worry about.

Consider these other alarming brain-related medical terms that doctors often toss out casually:

- **Mild cerebral atrophy** (as seen on an MRI): Translation: "It might be a sign of normal brain aging or the beginnings of a pathological condition." Indeed, imaging techniques are so sophisticated now that they almost always generate this kind of disconcerting "non-specific" information that may not mean anything at all.

- **Organic brain syndrome:** Translation: "We think you have Alzheimer's disease but aren't sure if something else is causing the problem (like alcohol abuse or a mini-stroke)."

The culprit is probably cortisol, a "stress" hormone produced by the adrenal glands. Stress, anxiety, pessimism, and depression all cause cortisol levels to soar. Particularly vulnerable is the brain's hippocampus, a region connected with learning and memory. Even short spikes in cortisol, such as before a big test, can cause temporary memory blips. However, a constant corrosive flood over time seems to bring on permanent shrinkage and atrophy—leading to memory loss. One study, for instance, found that women with a history of depression had smaller hippocampuses and scored lower on memory tests than non-depressed women, no matter what their age.[2] In fact, hippocampus shrinkage and diminished memory didn't seem to coincide with old age at all, but rather with the severity, duration, and frequency of depression.

Looking through a glass darkly may not explain your current memory problems. Nor does it guarantee later memory decline. Plenty of pessimists make it to

- **Chemical imbalance:** Translation: "You're probably depressed and will benefit from drugs."

- **TIA:** Translation: "You've had a transient ischemic attack or 'mini-stroke.'" Granted, TIAs aren't "real" strokes, but they do often warn of more serious strokes to come. Treating high blood pressure, heart disease, diabetes, and other risk factors can prevent further problems (see Chapter 6).

- **Bottom-line for patients:** If a diagnosis sounds vague or you don't understand what your doctor said, ask questions until you do. The Partnership for Clear Health Communication (www.askme3.org) recommends asking these three questions:
    1. What is my main problem?
    2. What do I need to do?
    3. Why is it important to do this?

- **Bottom-line for doctors:** Don't assume patients understand everything you say.
    1. Use plain language.
    2. Use visuals to illustrate a procedure or condition.
    3. Ask patients to "teach back" care instructions.

See Chapter 5 for more on cutting through medicalese and improving doctor-patient communications.

old age with their memories intact. But emotional factors are something to consider before assuming the worst about occasional cognitive misfires. Lower your stress, treat your depression, eliminate "glass-half-empty" thinking, and you might just feel the fog lift and your memory return.

HEADING OFF COGNITIVE DECLINE

It's a recurring theme in this book: what you eat, think, and do—in other words, how healthfully you live—can go a long way toward preventing disease. That goes for mental declines, as well. The following low-risk, high-benefit strategies certainly can't hurt and may actually prevent or halt cognitive problems before they escalate.

Eat Your Fruits and Veggies

Keeping artery-clogging saturated fat to a minimum and devouring plenty of antioxidant-rich fruits and vegetables is one of the best protections against fading cognitive powers.

The Technicolor diet described in Chapter 7 seems to confer the same benefits to the brain as it does against cancer. Antioxidants in phytonutrients (found in plant pigments) block certain biochemical changes in the aging brain caused by free-radical damage. Free radicals boost the number of "stress proteins," which ultimately impede memory.

Make sure to include a variety of intensely colored fruits and veggies at meals. Topping the list are blueberries and blackberries, rich in free-radical-fighting anthocyanins. Many other plant pigments contain mind-boosting nutrients, as well, including cranberries, strawberries, raspberries, kale, spinach, Brussels sprouts, alfalfa sprouts, and broccoli.

Enjoy an Occasional Glass of Wine

The much-touted, one-drink-a-day rule, so popular with heart experts, may also apply to the brain. The results of a large-scale study following more than 3,500 Japanese-American men for nearly twenty years, shows that moderate drinking (about one drink per day) during middle age can help preserve the brain's ability to think and reason later on.[3] Researchers started by recording how much the men drank during middle age, then measured their cognitive abilities eighteen years later. Those who enjoyed up to a drink a day tested higher than either the heavier drinkers or the non-drinkers. Men who drank four or more drinks per day scored lowest.

But Don't Smoke!

As if the pile of evidence against smoking weren't already sky-high, here's another one for the list. Smokers more than double their risk of developing Alzheimer's disease and vascular dementia (a common form caused by strokes, high blood pressure, and other vascular conditions) compared to non-smokers.

Get a Move On

Putter in the garden. Attend tai chi classes. Take a walk. Regular exercise significantly boosts your chances of warding off dementia, including Alzheimer's disease. And studies show that the more you use your body, the bigger the impact on your mental powers. One theory is that exercise actually produces neurons, which help the brain think and transmit signals.

Also important is variety, particularly among older people. Researchers observed more than 3,000 men and women over age sixty-five for eight years, tracking the kinds of activities they did—everything from household chores and hiking to swimming and bowling.[4] Those with the most wide-ranging exercise portfolios were far less likely to develop any type of dementia (except for individuals who were genetically predisposed to Alzheimer's disease). Variety may indeed be the spice of life—and the brain.

Control Blood Pressure

No matter what your age, high blood pressure (as well as obesity and high cholesterol) can hurt your brain's ability to function and may even contribute to the development of Alzheimer's disease and other dementias. Though the impact may not be as great among younger people with hypertension, one recent study shows that even eighteen year olds with elevated blood pressure are likely to notice some cognitive decline over time.[5]

Lowering your systolic measurement (the upper number) by 20 points and your diastolic pressure (the lower number) by 10 points could make all the difference. See Chapter 6 for more on blood pressure, cholesterol, and obesity.

Use It or Lose It

Exercising your mind is as crucial as exercising your body when it comes to staving off mental decline. And it may work the same way—by stimulating new brain cells. At least that's the consensus of several studies, showing that participating in regular, frequent leisure-time mind games helps older people not only halt memory lapses and cloudy thinking, but also significantly lower their risk of dementia. Best bets (every day, if possible): playing a musical instrument, reading, playing board games, doing crossword puzzles, and playing cards.

And Don't Forget Bedroom Games

Add a healthy sex life to your list of brain enhancers, as well. That's because sex releases a hormone called prolactin (found most commonly in pregnant women to help prepare their breasts for milk production). Its role isn't entirely understood, but it also seems to stimulate new brain cells.

TELL YOUR DOCTOR ABOUT THESE

Perhaps you're a little forgetful lately or worry that occasional "brain dead" moments signify something more serious. Discuss the following evidence-based, brain-enriching therapies with your doctor.

The B_{12} Connection

In the early twentieth century, researchers noted that certain individuals developed a mysterious form of anemia, dubbed "pernicious." They commonly suffered from weakness, tingling in their extremities, clumsiness, and an unsteady gait. Older patients sometimes appeared to have dementia or Alzheimer's disease.

In 1934, the Nobel Prize for medicine was awarded to George Whipple, George Minot, and William Murphy for their discovery that eating large quantities of raw liver helped people with pernicious anemia (previously thought to be an incurable condition).

In 1948, the key substance that gives liver its anemia-fighting ability—vitamin B_{12}—was isolated. People with pernicious anemia aren't able to adequately absorb vitamin B_{12} from their diet, so they need extra. Healthy people also need B_{12}, but because their bodies absorb it efficiently, a normal diet provides enough.

Since then, research has confirmed that many people, while not suffering full-blown pernicious anemia, nevertheless have a low-level B_{12} deficiency that can compromise mental performance and cause fatigue. As we'll see later in this chapter, B_{12} also boosts brain performance by working with other B vitamins to lower homocysteine (another possible risk factor for dementia and Alzheimer's disease).

I recommend getting tested for B_{12} deficiency (see Chapter 4), particularly if you're feeling fatigued or your memory is sub-optimal. Consider supplementing if your B_{12} levels are below 400 picograms per milliliter (the ordinary cut-off for outright deficiency is 200 pg/ml or less). Try B_{12} shots or take 500–1,000 micrograms (mcg) of B_{12} daily. Dissolving the tablet under your tongue (sublingually) might help absorption, but this isn't thoroughly established.

Blood Sugar

My patient Sally is a classic example of how blood sugar problems can compromise mental efficiency. I began to suspect hypoglycemia after she told me her concentration typically bottomed out in mid-morning, after a typical breakfast of cornflakes and skim milk, and again in the afternoon after lunch. I performed an oral glucose tolerance test, and three hours after ingesting the sugar challenge, sure enough, Sally's blood sugar plunged and she became barely coherent and shaky.

Hypoglycemia literally starves the brain of glucose energy (essential for full brain function). Most conventional doctors believe hypoglycemia is rare, but it's actually fairly prevalent. The brain is a hungry, rapidly metabolizing organ. At rest, it consumes one-third of the body's total glucose requirement (glucose is converted from carbohydrates). Fuel shortages there create an array of symptoms, including problems in concentration, memory and mood, spaciness, fatigue, sugar craving, headaches, depression, and panic attacks.

To understand why, it helps to understand that all carbs aren't created equal; their rate of conversion to sugar depends on their complexity. Complex carbohydrates like beans, provide a slow time-release of sugar because it's contained in complex molecules of starch interwoven with fiber. However, sugars and refined carbohydrates (foods made from white flour) provide a rapid sugar fix (that familiar sugar high).

Unfortunately, "what goes up must come down"—sometimes with a dizzying crash. The surge of glucose prompts the body to summon its insulin reserves and swiftly contain the flood. The rapid decline in glucose triggers extreme hunger—especially carbohydrate craving—and the brain becomes starved for its preferred fuel, glucose. When that happens, you feel brain dead!

Studies show that even mild hypoglycemia can alter brain function. If you suspect blood sugar fluctuations, have your doctor give you an oral glucose tolerance test, which more precisely pinpoints minute dips in blood glucose that standard tests may miss (see Chapter 4). The test also better detects insulin spikes that can occur after eating carbohydrates—a possible sign of Syndrome X (discussed later in this section).

And don't forget to look at the timing of meals. One study of older people, ages sixty-one to seventy, found that consuming calories after an overnight fast boosted their memory test scores.[6] Mom was right all along: breakfast may be the most important meal of the day.

Drugs or Dementia?

Conventional medicine's approach to aging often means throwing drugs at older patients rather than dealing holistically with their growing number of medical maladies. One aspect of a holistic approach is being mindful of potential brain-numbing drug side effects.

The fact is, many drugs prescribed to older patients—and even a few available over the counter—can cause temporary memory and concentration lapses, and may even be mistaken for the beginnings of dementia. Mental problems are often heightened by adverse interactions that can occur when several drugs are used simultaneously or when certain medications are misused or overused (such as sleeping pills or tranquilizers). The result? Doctors end up prescribing even more drugs to counteract these drug-induced cognitive declines.

Many medications used to treat Parkinson's disease, depression, allergies, migraine, and irritable bowel syndrome can cause these "anticholinergic" side effects. These include dementia-like symptoms, like memory loss, disorientation and confusion, as well as dry mouth, constipation, dizziness, and rapid heartbeat.

OTC (over-the-counter) drugs with potential anticholinergic effects include remedies for indigestion, such as Tagamet, Pepcid, and Zantac, as well as cold and flu treatments and hay fever medications.

If your thinking is cloudy since going on one or more medications, talk to your doctor about using natural alternatives. Lowering your dosage of "culprit" drugs or halting them altogether usually reverses dementia-like symptoms.

Essential Fatty Acids

That schoolyard bully who called you a "fat head" wasn't so far off the mark. Your brain is made up of fat—in fact, it's about 60 percent fat. And not just any fat. It contains more essential fatty acids (mostly omega-3s and some omega-6s) than any other organ in your body. These fats are the building blocks of cell membranes in the brain, as well as myelin, the fatty insulating sheath surrounding nerve fibers that help carry messages faster.

In the brain's case, you literally are what you eat. For optimum brain function, cut out saturated fats and trans fats (these "bad" fats degrade your brain) and add plenty of omega-3s, including fish oil. That means forgoing processed crackers, packaged snacks and fried foods, and adding more cold-water fish, nuts, and flaxseeds. Also consider following a heart-healthy diet (what's good for the heart also seems to be good for the brain). Take two 1,000-milligram (mg) fish oil capsules per day containing 420 mg of the fatty acid EPA (eicosapentaenoic acid) and 300 mg of DHA (docosahexaenoic acid). See Chapter 6 for more on a heart-boosting diet, EFAs, and fish oil.

The Iron Connection

Iron is vital for the production of hemoglobin, which helps red blood cells carry oxygen to the brain and other parts of the body. Insufficient iron can lead to another kind of brain-altering anemia. And even modest iron deficiencies can lead to fatigue and weakness, as well as diminished memory, attention, and ability to learn.

Have your doctor test your iron levels using a ferritin test (see Chapter 4). Many "natural" iron formulations are too weak to pack a punch. I recommend a newer prescription form of iron called Niferex. Take 150 mg two or three times a day. Iron is best absorbed with additional vitamin C (500 mg three times daily). For those who can't tolerate supplemental iron, try a diet high in iron-rich foods, including red meat and organ meat (the best sources of more bio-available heme iron), beans, green leafy vegetables, dried fruits, nuts, and whole grain breads.

Magnesium

Your middle-age memory lapses may also be helped with extra magnesium. Studies show that magnesium helps regulate an important brain receptor that aids in learning and memory (the NMDA receptor). Unfortunately, many of us don't get enough magnesium. Deficiencies can result in diminished cognitive function at any age. To prevent or reverse memory problems, eat plenty of magnesium-rich foods (dark green leafy vegetables, nuts, and legumes) and take 400 mg of magnesium daily.

Meditation

Given the degrading impact of cortisol on the brain, anything that lessens stress is likely to improve your mental powers. Meditation is a natural, drugless antidote to the mind-numbing pace and worries of modern life. Just fifteen to twenty minutes in the morning and evening has been shown to not only diminish the ravages of stress on the body, but boost intelligence, creativity, learning, memory, and reasoning. Learn more about Transcendental Meditation's mind-boosting benefits at www.tm.org. (See Chapter 6 for more on meditation techniques.)

Syndrome X

While you're rethinking meals and managing blood sugar, you might also consider a little old-fashioned weight loss. As noted in previous chapters, insulin resistance (a.k.a. Syndrome X) puts people at risk for heart disease, cancer and many other maladies. Now research suggests that insulin resistance and accompanying inflammation may also contribute to memory loss and possibly even Alzheimer's disease.[7] The tell-tale signs of Syndrome X are high blood pressure, high cholesterol, high blood sugar, and a large belly (see Chapters 6 and 7).

And consider this: There's a possible third type of diabetes that may be connected to Alzheimer's disease.[8] Researchers have discovered that insulin isn't just produced in the pancreas, but also in the brain, and that it's necessary for survival of brain cells. Like type 1 and type 2 diabetes, type 3 begins with insulin-production problems. As the problem worsens, brain cells begin to degenerate. In fact, researchers have discovered that insulin production in the brain of Alzheimer's patients is severely curtailed, particularly in areas most affected by the disease, such as the hippocampus.

REVISITING CONTROVERSIES

The following therapies may help prevent or fend off cognitive problems, but they remain controversial. Even so, you may want to discuss them with your doctor.

Role of Hormones

The brain requires youthful levels of certain hormones to facilitate cell energy metabolism, maintain proper levels of acetylcholine (a key neurotransmitter that aids in memory), and protect brain-cell membrane function. In my opinion, aging people often require some hormone replacement therapy (HRT) for optimum brain functioning. However, recent controversies over HRT have left many patients gun-shy—many of whom could truly benefit from taking the right hormones.

Estrogen

Time was when women routinely turned to estrogen replacement therapy to help relieve their menopausal symptoms, including that "brain dead" feeling. Indeed, science suggests that estrogen plays a significant role in cognition. The brain is actually loaded with estrogen receptors located in several key areas that facilitate memory (including the hippocampus).

However, many women and doctors are now spooked by the thought of using estrogen. Another problem: research on estrogen's braining-boosting powers, particularly in postmenopausal women, is contradictory. While some studies show that taking it after menopause improves memory and other brain functions—and may even protect against Alzheimer's disease—others show no benefit at all. A few even suggest a negative effect.

The confusion, however, may result from poor study design, plus the fact that many studies used synthetic estrogen rather than bio-identical forms that more closely mimic human estrogen (see Chapter 3 for more on interpreting study results). In other words, I don't think that we can draw definitive conclusions without better, more targeted studies.

Bottom-line: As with heart disease, I don't advise taking hormones after normal menopause unless you're suffering from severe symptoms. However, many women, including my patient Sally, have found that HRT helps their menopause-related memory slips. In Sally's case, I prescribed bio-identical estrogen and progesterone, balanced with DHEA and testosterone (see next) to help restore her equanimity and focus. I prefer formulations from compounding pharmacies that specialize in customized natural HRT therapies, such as College Pharmacy or Women's International Pharmacy (see Resources for Patients). Practitioners familiar with prescribing natural hormones may be found on the American College for Advancement in Medicine's website (www.acam.org).

A corollary to the estrogen story is soy. Contradictory study results abound here, as well. While some show that adding soy isoflavones to your diet (which may mimic the effects of estrogen in the brain without the adverse effects of HRT) can significantly improve cognition, others show the opposite effect.

Bottom-line: I believe soy has a place among brain-boosting foods. I prefer food sources and not soy supplements. The best, least-refined sources are cooked soybeans (edamame), tofu, and tempeh. Try two to three 4–6 ounce servings of these foods per week.

Testosterone

Age-related declines in testosterone are linked to forgetfulness, not just in men but also in women (who produce the hormone in smaller amounts). Evidence suggests that offering testosterone replacement therapy to both men and women may halt some memory losses.

However, like estrogen, the idea of supplementing with testosterone is still highly controversial, particularly for women. Even so, I've seen it work wonders (as in Sally's case).

Whether you're a man or woman, I recommend having your testosterone levels tested (see Chapter 4). If an imbalance is uncovered, speak to your doctor about taking natural testosterone. I prefer prescription topical testosterone in absorbable cream form made by a compounding pharmacy. Women should take 2–10 mg per day. Men should take 50–200 mg per day.

DHEA

Often over-hyped as a fountain of youth, DHEA (dehydroepiandrosterone) is nonetheless a vital hormone involved in several important bodily functions, including improving brain cell activity and enhancing memory. As we age, however, daily production of DHEA drops—from 30 mg at age twenty to less than 6 mg at age eighty. Several studies have linked flagging DHEA levels to the onset of disease, including Alzheimer's. But its use remains controversial.

I'm a big proponent of DHEA, and have found appropriate doses (given after testing for deficiency) an indispensable tool for sharpening mental acuity and offsetting mild depression and inertia (see Chapter 4).

DHEA is available over the counter, but I don't recommend it for those under twenty-one, pregnant women, or those recovering from prostate or breast cancer. Seek out a physician knowledgeable in DHEA administration. For women, I recommend 5–25 mg per day; for men, 25–50 mg daily.

Thyroid

A thyroid hormone deficiency may also result in poor brain function, including problems with concentration, memory disturbances, and depression. Unfortunately, many physicians attribute these symptoms to other health problems and never think to test for low thyroid function. And even when they do, patients may not be properly diagnosed because test results come back "normal."

"Normal" is simply a range that most healthy people fall into. It's not one-size-fits-all. Some people with normal results are actually deficient. Talk to your doctor about getting a complete panel of thyroid blood tests rather than just the more common TSH test (thyroid stimulating hormone).

Mercury, Lead, and Chemicals

As we saw in Chapter 4, environmental toxins—particularly heavy metals and synthetic chemicals used in everyday products—can ravage the body over time. That includes the brain. In fact, these byproducts of modern life (which show up in abundance in most people when tested) may actually play a role in age-related cognitive impairment and even Alzheimer's disease.

The problem, though, is that most conventional physicians don't think to test for them. Even when they do offer standard blood tests, results tend to reveal only very high levels of toxic metals (not other chemicals) in the blood and don't tell how much is stored in tissues. That's why I recommend a "provocative chelation" test (see Chapter 4).

Unfortunately, testing for the thousands of other non-metal chemicals that contaminate our air, water, and food is more difficult because many states don't permit it. Check with your doctor about availability of testing in your area. See my book *Intelligent Medicine* for more on body-burden testing.

Antioxidants

As noted in previous chapters, many antioxidants, like vitamin E, are currently under the gun for either having no effect on diseases of aging or for actually speeding up their deadly effects. The same goes for cognitive problems, including Alzheimer's disease.

Vitamins E and C

Many brain disorders, like Alzheimer's and Parkinson's disease, appear to originate with oxidative stress and inflammation in the body. For this reason, researchers have looked to antioxidants, particularly vitamin E with its potent free-radical-fighting abilities, as a possible safeguard against brain disorders and age-related declines.

In fact, studies show that it may lower the risk of Parkinson's when taken in moderate to high doses. And when combined with higher doses of vitamin C, it appears to significantly reduce the chance that someone will develop Alzheimer's disease later in life.

That's the good news. The bad news is that not all studies support this idea.

While I agree that more studies are needed, I don't think we should ignore the significant body of existing research showing that vitamins E and C and other antioxidants may be important components of a brain-boosting strategy. I recommend 400–800 international units (IU) per day of natural vitamin E (mixed tocopherols with tocotrienols) and 500 mg of Ester C (an easier form to absorb), two to three times daily.

Coenzyme Q_{10}

Coenzyme Q_{10} isn't exactly on the radar of conventional medicine—and certainly not front and center in the field of brain research—at least not yet. However, a growing number of studies suggest its antioxidant properties may protect the brain against free-radical damage and boost learning power, particularly when combined with vitamin E. Research also shows that it may safeguard against neurodegenerative diseases, including Parkinson's disease, Huntington's disease, and ALS (amyotrophic lateral sclerosis or Lou Gehrig's disease).

For prevention, take 150 mg of CoQ_{10} daily. Patients with Parkinson's, Alzheimer's, or other serious brain disorders may require as much as 1,200–1,600 mg per day (see Resources for Patients for more information).

Alpha-Lipoic Acid

This antioxidant is unique in its ability to cross the blood-brain barrier, which can hinder other antioxidants from reaching brain cells. Alpha-lipoic acid quenches free radicals and seems to have a special affinity for repairing neurons, as indicated by its status as a medication in Germany for treating diabetic nerve degeneration. Take 200–300 mg twice daily.

Herbal and Nutritional Supplements

The jury is still out on the effectiveness of these herbs and nutritional supplements for cognitive problems. Nevertheless, some evidence suggests they may be useful.

Ginkgo Biloba

You've probably seen over-the-counter ginkgo supplements claiming to improve memory and concentration. Indeed, hundreds of European studies and some in the United States provide strong evidence that ginkgo boosts memory and mental acuity in healthy adults, possibly by improving blood flow to the brain and via its antioxidant effect. Other studies support its use in slowing the progression of Alzheimer's disease. In fact, in Europe, ginkgo has long been used for treating dementia and other brain disorders.

However, controversy continues over the quality and validity of many of these studies. What's more, other studies, published in prestigious journals, show the opposite effect—mainly that ginkgo has no impact on Alzheimer's and does little to enhance brain function in healthy adults.

Even so, I think the evidence that ginkgo improves memory, thinking, and learning (in those with Alzheimer's disease and those without) remains promising. Better studies, which are currently underway, should tell us more.

In the meantime, discuss taking ginkgo with your doctor. Because many OTC brands vary widely in quality and amount of active ingredients, I recommend a standardized ginkgo biloba extract containing at least 24% flavone glycosides and 6% terpene lactones. To enhance memory and mental performance, try 120 mg daily, divided into two doses. For Alzheimer's and other dementias, take up to 240 mg a day, divided into two doses. Because of ginkgo's anti-clotting properties don't combine with aspirin or anticoagulants, such as Coumadin.

Ginseng

Like ginkgo, this ancient herb—long used in Asia as an energy tonic—looks promising for treatment of various dementias, including Alzheimer's disease, and vascular dementia. However, research results remain contradictory.

Even so, I believe ginseng is worth considering for its brain-boosting effects. Though researchers don't yet understand which substances in ginseng are at work, one new study, funded by the National Institutes of Health, recently made some headway. Using American ginseng, researchers found that a partially purified extract of some of the herb's active chemicals, called ginsenosides, helped fight degeneration in the brains of rats (similar to the damage found in Parkinson's disease) better than a whole-root preparation.[9] And Chinese research has shown ginseng facilitates brain recovery in stroke patients. More research should help clarify which components of ginseng are most effective.

For cognitive enhancement, I prefer *Panax ginseng* from Korea or China to Siberian or American ginseng. Because ginseng formulations are so variable and aren't yet standardized, I recommend the raw root, obtained from a reliable herbal apothecary. Take 1–2 grams of root per day for up to three months.

Curcumin

Scientists originally singled out curcumin—an extract of the herb turmeric that gives curry its yellow color—after it was noted that Alzheimer's disease is rare in India where the spice is nearly a dietary staple. Since then, hunch has turned into promising reality. Research on rats has found that curcumin activates an enzyme in the brain that defends it against free-radical oxidation.

Curcumin also appears to slow the effects of Alzheimer's disease and other neurodegenerative diseases in mice by reducing inflammation in the brain and blocking the accumulation of beta-amyloid plaques, sticky substances that cause

Alzheimer's.[10] More studies are now underway to see if curcumin also protects against Alzheimer's disease in humans.

Your doctor may not think to prescribe any of the yellow stuff, but I recommend it as part of a brain-boosting regimen. For prevention, take one or two 500-mg capsules daily with food; for more advanced neurodegenerative conditions, take four to six capsules per day (see Resources for Patients).

Creatine

Produced naturally in the liver, kidneys, and pancreas, you may recognize this amino acid as something athletes pop to enhance their physical endurance. Again, research is nowhere complete, but early evidence suggests creatine may also boost brain function as well—and with few side effects. The usual dosage is 5 grams (around 1 teaspoon of creatine powder) once daily.

PS (phosphatidylserine) and PC (phosphatidylcholine)

Derived from lecithin, PS and PC are both phospholipids found in the cell membranes of brain neurons. PC is a building block of the neurotransmitter acetylcholine, and PS is the dominant phospholipid that makes up brain cell membranes. Unfortunately, both decline with age.

Research is contradictory on whether PC and PS actually act as "brain food," but supplementing may offer a cognitive boost, particularly if you don't eat a lot of high-phospholipid foods, like soy, eggs, and the brain tissue of animals.

One novel approach to phospholipid replacement involves a newly developed formula called NT Factor, which combines a wide spectrum of phospholipids critical to membrane function. Research suggests that NT Factor may enhance brain metabolism by improving the efficiency of mitochondria, the cell structures responsible for energy production in the brain and throughout the body. I recommend two capsules twice daily (see Resources for Patients).

Vinpocetine

A circulatory enhancer derived from the periwinkle plant, research shows that vinpocetine improves oxygen uptake in critical brain areas linked to cognition and memory. It's also sometimes touted as a remedy for tinnitus and mild hearing loss. Suggested dosage: 5–10 mg once or twice daily.

Huperzine A

Extracted from the herb "toothed clubmoss" (used in Chinese medicine), huperzine is believed to increase acetylcholine levels by halting its breakdown in the brain. Take 150–200 mg twice daily. However, use caution when combining it with standard Alzheimer's drugs, since it may negatively enhance their effects.

DMAE

A naturally occurring compound found in the brain, DMAE, or dimethy-laminoethanol, has long been touted as an aid in memory and cognition. Evidence shows it may increase levels of choline, a building block for acetylcholine. Take 75–100 mg twice daily.

Acetyl-L-Carnitine

Research on the role of this important amino acid has been ongoing for nearly twenty-five years. And, like so much research, study results are a mixed bag, particularly with regard to the brain. It's widely accepted that acetyl-L-carnitine enhances energy production in brain cells and promotes production of acetyl-choline. Indeed, several small, double-blind studies show that it delays the progression of Alzheimer's disease and may slow cognitive declines in healthy older people. However, a few larger studies have failed to replicate these findings, possibly because of differing methodologies.

Nevertheless, I recommend taking two to four 500-mg acetyl-L-carnitine capsules daily on an empty stomach with water or juice (preferably forty-five minutes before breakfast and lunch). Because it may have a stimulating effect, avoid taking it in the evening.

Celiac Disease

Only recently have doctors begun to fully understand the myriad ways celiac disease can manifest itself in the body. That's probably why mainstream medicine has yet to connect all the dots between gluten sensitivity and brain malfunctions.

Here's how it works. For people with celiac disease, gluten (found in wheat, rye, and other grains) actually damages their intestines and prevents them from taking in important nutrients. Over time, this deprivation may damage every major organ in the body, including the brain.

In fact, neurological disorders, such as early-onset dementia, are found in about 10 percent of celiac sufferers. A recent Italian study, for instance, discovered that nearly 75 percent of patients with untreated celiac disease had at least one hypoperfused region in their brain—meaning blood vessel damage.[11] Only one patient on a gluten-free diet and none of the celiac-free subjects had such damage. In addition, blood flow was lower in many brain areas of untreated patients compared to treated patients and the control group.

If you suspect celiac disease, ask your doctor to give you an anti-gliadin antibody test (see Chapter 4).

Neurotransmitters

These substances (including dopamine, adrenaline, and acetylcholine) help send nerve impulses across brain synapses. However, because of stress and aging, neurotransmitter levels often decline over time. The result can be fatigue, depression or anxiety, sleep problems, sugar cravings, and lack of mental acuity.

If you suspect a deficiency, have your doctor test your neurotransmitter levels (see Chapter 4). Imbalances may require supplementing with amino acids (neurotransmitter building blocks), like tyrosine, and 5-HTP (5-hydroxytryptophan), or with co-factors for neurotransmitter synthesis, like vitamins B_5 and B_6. Unfortunately, there's no "cookbook" for addressing individual neurotransmitter imbalances, so consult a practitioner who is well versed in this approach.

Homocysteine

In Chapter 6 we saw that high blood levels of homocysteine (an amino acid) is believed to promote atherosclerosis and boost risk of heart disease. Taking folic acid and other B vitamins (particularly B_6 and B_{12}) helps break down homocysteine, but at this time the effect on heart attack and stroke risk is unclear. Interestingly, studies also point to a link between high homocysteine/low B vitamin levels and vascular dementia and Alzheimer's disease.

However, early evidence doesn't yet support treating cognitive impairment by supplementing with B vitamins to normalize homocysteine levels. Keep in mind, though, that most studies have only looked at short-term supplementation. More research is needed on the impact of taking B vitamins for longer periods.

In the meantime, I recommend testing for homocysteine (see Chapter 4) and a good B vitamin regimen for brain health. Ten micromoles of homocysteine per liter of blood is considered good, but I prefer to go even lower to 8 micromoles per liter. If your homocysteine is high, take 50 mg of B_6 once or twice daily; 500–1,000 mcg of B_{12} per day; and 800 mcg of folic acid daily. Some patients with very high–homocysteine levels may require higher doses.

As we've seen, aging needn't inevitably lead to cognitive declines or dementia. Any number of other factors can masquerade as memory problems and even the beginnings of Alzheimer's disease, including emotional distress, depression, poor diet, lack of exercise, nutrient deficiencies, underlying health problems and hormonal imbalances. In many instances, treating cognitive problems simply requires recognizing what's really happening in the body and making the necessary adjustments via dietary changes, nutritional supplements, and other CAM therapies rather than employing heavy-hitting conventional treatments.

In the next chapter, we'll examine other "diseases" that also sometimes result from underlying dietary, emotional, and hormonal imbalances, or simply from natural changes that accompany aging. Indeed, many of these conditions are now considered "bona fide" diseases with a slew of powerful mainstream drugs available to treat them. But as we'll see, CAM therapies are often preferable.

Dealing with Diseases
That Aren't Diseases

Doctor, doctor I'm begging on my knees
Won't you tell me please
What could be my malady?

—THE JAMES BARCLAY HARVEST

Consider the options available to people facing midlife. Even if they don't suffer from an overt disease, they're likely to be handed a prescription or urged to undergo surgery to "fix" even minor ailments. If their blood pressure isn't yet high, but creeping up, they might be dubbed pre-hypertensive and placed on "light" medication, including a statin drug and daily aspirin.

If they're female, they probably have a touch of osteopenia (pre-osteoporosis), prompting another prescription for bone-strengthening drugs. And for those with a family history of breast cancer or lumpy breasts, their doctor might even consider a powerful hormone blocker.

Men concerned about receding hairlines now have Propecia. And just in case sexual performance isn't up to par, a slew of erectile dysfunction drugs are available for the taking.

Likewise, there are antidepressants and anti-anxiety drugs for occasional mood blips; attention-focusing drugs for "spaciness" and low productivity (a.k.a. "Adult Attention Deficit Disorder"); a plethora of antihistamines for seasonal allergies; and powerful acid blockers to "cure" occasional indigestion resulting from poor diet. And, of course, researchers are anxiously seeking the Holy Grail of modern pharmaceuticals: a pill that curbs appetite and helps burn fat effortlessly—all without side effects!

Indeed, the possibilities are endless . . .

But do these conditions really warrant treatment? A recent issue of the *British Medical Journal* decries the "medicalization" of common complaints.[1] With most truly sick people already on prescription drugs, pharmaceutical companies have begun looking elsewhere for additional profits. Their answer? Create new "disease" niches (mostly mild, ubiquitous ailments) and market preventive "lifestyle drugs" to ward them off. Indeed, catering to the droves of "worried well" is far more lucrative than selling drugs to the few who really need them.

A prime example is "FSD"—the new acronym for "female sexual dysfunction." Is this really a new disorder or merely an effort to keep pace with men in the race toward sexual fulfillment? Is there really a hormone fix for women's flagging libidos? Or are we simply searching for something that can't be cured in a bottle—including relationship ills that arise from unfulfilled romantic longings or lack of respect?

Unfortunately, our endless quest for "cures" only fans fears and dissatisfaction. By endlessly pointing out what could happen, otherwise healthy people begin worrying about future diseases—even believing they have them or soon will. Offer them a "panacea" and expectations soar.

Even old drugs suddenly find new life as demand for perfect health skyrockets. Witness the antidepressant Effexor, recently covertly marketed to doctors as a cure for "shopaholism" after a small study demonstrated it curbed buying binges. Paxil now has approval to treat shyness (newly branded as "social phobia"), and Prozac, which became a cheap generic after its patent expired, has been revived as Serafem, a new treatment for premenstrual dysphoria (severe PMS). Even aging itself is now considered curable, or at the very least something to delay indefinitely.

Unfortunately, you don't have to be Tom Cruise to suspect that things are a little out of hand! (Cruise recently garnered attention for lambasting the widespread use of drugs to treat conditions such as depression.) Indeed, many health problems are simply natural changes in the body from aging. Others are minor complaints that don't really warrant major pharmaceutical treatment or invasive surgery (akin to removing tough stains with powerful acids when a little baking soda and vinegar will do). Or they're harbingers of more serious conditions in the making that can be easily corrected via lifestyle changes.

In this chapter we'll look at some of these diseases that aren't really diseases. We'll examine what can happen when patients are over-medicated and over-treated for problems that may not require such drastic measures. We'll also look at gentler, more natural approaches to these conditions, as well as how patients can work with their doctors to avoid "medicalizing" every health problem.

OVER-DIAGNOSED AND OVER-PRESCRIBED

Ben was a twenty-nine-year-old stockbroker who came to the Hoffman Center complaining of severe GERD (gastroesophageal reflux disease), a "backflow" of stomach acid into the esophagus that causes discomfort and more severe problems. Despite receiving a powerful acid blocker from his gastroenterologist, Ben was often nauseated and bloated, and suffered from chest pains.

Because the usual medications weren't helping, his doctor recommended additional tests, which revealed a hiatal hernia that was allowing food to backflow from his stomach into his esophagus. His doctor recommended a procedure called fundoplication. This involves constructing a new "valve" between the esophagus and the stomach by wrapping the upper portion of the stomach (the fundus) around the lowest part of the esophagus. The surgery can be done laparoscopically via special robot arms inserted into tiny incisions in the patient's abdomen and chest.

Because Ben wasn't sure he wanted surgery, he came to me. I agreed he should proceed with caution, but noted that many patients with hard-to-relieve reflux get substantial relief from surgery. However, I added that a small but significant percentage don't get better with fundoplication, and many who do get relief must remain on acid-blockers for life. Not only that but the potential for complications is also high, including difficulty swallowing (dysphagia), a feeling of fullness, flatulence, and diarrhea. And as I explained, fundoplication may be nothing more than the latest surgical fix-of-choice (after supplanting ulcer surgery in the mid-1990s). My fear was—and is—that many patients who don't find relief from acid-blocking drugs are automatically fed into the fundoplication pipeline with little consideration for other options.

Ben and I finally agreed he should try natural interventions before turning to surgery. I offered no guarantees because many serious cases of GERD are beyond alternative fixes, and I suggested that he remain on acid blockers for the time being.

Ben had already opted for a better diet. Even though it hadn't helped much, it was a good start. Gone were his beloved steaks, burgers, omelets, and chicken wings, replaced by low-fat meals, including high-fiber cereal, soymilk, fish, chicken, salad, brown rice, and low-fat cheese. He'd even sworn off candy and was now consuming lots of fruit, including nutritious trail mix for afternoon snacks. Unfortunately, he still needed more nutritional guidance.

I ordered a panel of tests on Ben, then sent him down the hall to our nutritionist for detailed instructions on our GERD diet. We urge patients to avoid the usual suspects—coffee, chocolate, alcohol, fried foods, tomato sauce, carbonated beverages—but also go a step further by recommending that they also shun simple sugars, excess fruits and juices, and fermentable starches like breads and whole grains. My intuition told me that Ben's problem was not so much a "bum" valve, but rather that his stomach had become a fermenting vat. Ben had tried to eat right, but was inadvertently pouring natural sugars and hard-to-digest starches into a confined chamber where gas-producing bacteria and yeasts were happily proliferating. The resulting volatile mix had turned his esophagus into Vesuvius!

When Ben's tests came back there were additional surprises. Since he was young and looked relatively slim, no one had paid attention to his cardiovascular

risk. Not only had his father suffered a heart attack at age fifty, but Ben's cholesterol was over 200 and his beneficial HDL was far too low at 35. Moreover, his
triglycerides were running neck and neck with his cholesterol, suggesting that he
had a case of insulin resistance, or Syndrome X. Sure enough, when the results of
his glucose tolerance test came in, Ben showed serious blood sugar spikes and an
elevated insulin response to the sugar challenge. His carb-rich diet had only been
feeding the problem.

Additionally Ben's allergy tests came back positive for wheat, dairy, and
corn—foods that we'd already suggested he avoid on the trial GERD diet. He also
admitted that he'd gained fifteen pounds since college due to inactivity. I suggested he get back to exercising and lose some weight.

After three weeks, Ben showed a distinct improvement, though he still had
occasional pain, bloating, and fullness. The DGL (deglycyrrhizinated licorice)
lozenges we'd given him on his first visit (discussed later in this chapter) were
soothing his esophagus, and he was faithfully taking the probiotic pills we had
prescribed.

Within six months, Ben's gastrointestinal problems were all but gone. Not
only didn't he need surgery, but also, as I was delighted to learn, he'd successfully
tapered his drugs. Moreover, he looked and felt great, with more energy than he'd
had in years. After shedding pounds of flab, he was now playing basketball and
swimming several days a week. And sure enough, his cholesterol had come down
dramatically—to an ideal 150 with HDL of 45 and triglycerides of 90.

OUT OF WHACK

Medicine has a somewhat schizophrenic take on "disease." Most of us, including
health professionals, tend to think of diseases as discrete entities that fit neatly into
clear categories. In other words, symptoms A, B, and C mean you have Disease Z.

But that's not really true. Current disease definitions describe ideal scenar-
ios—usually hammered out by a consensus of medical experts. What's more, they
often change. With cholesterol, for instance, better statins have led the medical
establishment to move its cholesterol goal posts. What was once considered "normal" is now considered "borderline" high!

All this is a far cry from the origin of the word "dis-ease," meaning a depar-
ture from wellness that causes suffering, whether or not it's fatal. Most daily complaints don't fit into these ideal disease categories. For one thing, many health
conditions mimic other conditions, resulting in misdiagnosis (for example,
depressed patients often complain of pain and lethargy, which can look like
chronic fatigue syndrome). The fact is health is messy, and the rising number of
health problems (resulting from raised wellness expectations) increasingly eludes
diagnosis.

Ben is a good example. His GERD turned out to be something else entirely—a problem caused by a diet that was inappropriate for his digestive system and metabolism. Unfortunately, Ben's doctor had medicalized his digestive trouble, labeling it a "disease" and almost landing him in the surgery suite. And because his Syndrome X and other heart risks were never uncovered, sooner or later Ben would have ended up with a real disease, requiring diabetes and antihypertensive drugs and possibly even heart surgery.

Thankfully, Ben chose to optimize his health using natural approaches rather than face a lifetime of medicalization. Unfortunately, many patients aren't so lucky. They languish in the medical system for years as doctors attempt to diagnose and treat them for conditions they either don't have, like Ben, or ones that may not require potent interventions.

Even doctors who might prefer a less aggressive approach to "disease-fighting" are reluctant to flout conventional medical wisdom. For one thing, they fear being sued for malpractice. "Watchful waiting" may be preferable (as in certain cases of prostate cancer, transient mood disorders, back pain, and menopausal symptoms). Or a lighter hand, using natural and low-tech complementary thera-

PRACTICE TIP: PATIENT INFLUENCE

Patients who request prescription drugs during visits to their doctor are more likely to receive them than those who remain mum, according to a new study in the *Journal of the American Medical Association*.[2] Researchers sent actors pretending to be patients into 152 doctors' offices to see if they could get prescriptions. One group of patients simulated major depression (characterized by lethargy, difficulty sleeping, and long periods of sadness), while the other pretended to have "adjustment disorder with depressed mood" brought on by career problems (a condition that doesn't usually warrant use of antidepressants). In both groups, one-third asked for a specific antidepressant (Paxil), one-third made a general request for any antidepressant, and the final one-third didn't request anything.

Most interesting were the results for the adjustment disorder group. Those who requested Paxil were five times more likely to get a prescription (even though their symptoms didn't warrant such treatment) than those who didn't request any drugs (55 percent versus 10 percent). In the depressed group, 53 percent got Paxil after asking for it versus 31 percent who didn't request an antidepressant. Bottom-line: Direct-to-consumer drug ads may be prompting patients to ask for more prescriptions, and doctors may be unduly or inappropriately influenced by these requests.

pies, may work wonders—particularly for conditions that only pose danger years from now. But most physicians are inclined to find and treat something—anything—rather than risk inaction or the appearance of practicing substandard care. Plus, patients often push for drug treatments they read or hear about in ads (see "Practice Tip: Patient Influence" on page 177). Besides, there's little financial incentive for holding off treatment. Ours is a system that rewards decisive and dramatic intervention—even when there's doubt—and asks questions later.

The following section looks at several "diseases" that are increasingly targeted with high-tech drugs and surgery. We'll cover natural, constructive interventions that may forestall or relieve these conditions without significant risk or expense. We'll also look at ways to get buy-in from your doctor (see "Changing Directions Midstream: Backing Off Conventional Treatments" on page 180).

Chronic Fatigue Syndrome (CFS)

CFS is actually a bone fide disease with strict criteria defined by the Centers for Disease Control. Many sufferers complain that calling it chronic fatigue syndrome trivializes the suffering and disability they experience on a daily basis, which goes way beyond just being tired. In fact, so many patients have consulted me over the years for CFS (or its lesser manifestations, like exhaustion and debilitation) that I wrote a book in 1991 entitled *Tired All the Time: How to Regain Your Lost Energy*. In it, I detail how to troubleshoot hidden problems and the many natural interventions that have lifted my patients' exhaustion over the years. Among them:

- **Check thyroid function:** Even where thyroid function tests indicate that patients are in the normal range, natural thyroid extract (Armour Thyroid, Euthroid, etc.) can often restore energy. See www.thyroid-info.com, or read *Living Well with Hypothyroidism,* by Mary Shomon. Hidden hypothyroidism (sluggish thyroid) should be considered, particularly when fatigue is accompanied by inability to lose weight, dry skin, coldness, and, in women, heavy periods/PMS.

- **Mitochondrial support:** Mitochondria help power cells, converting energy into usable forms. Some researchers believe that CFS is partly a disease of mitochondrial dysfunction. Nutrients that support the mitochondria include:

  - Carnitine: Take 500–1,000 milligrams (mg) three times daily.

  - Coenzyme Q_{10}: Take 300–1,600 mg daily.

  - NADH (ENADA): Nicotinamide adenine dinucleotide is a coenzyme made from an activated form of vitamin B_3, or niacin, that helps cells extract energy from nutrients. Take 5–10 mg twice daily.

  - Propax with NT Factor: Take one packet twice daily.

  - Riboflavin: Take 50–200 mg twice daily.

- **Neurotransmitters:** Maybe the problem is all in your head? But that doesn't mean you're imagining it. Low levels of neurotransmitters in the brain (chemicals like serotonin, dopamine, norepinephrine, and GABA) are associated with exhaustion. Get your neurotransmitters checked under the guidance of a nutritionally oriented health professional (see Chapter 4). If low, consider supplementing with amino acids (neurotransmitter building blocks), such as L-tyrosine and 5-HTP (5-hydroxytryptophan), as well as vitamin B_6.

- **Check for low iron, B_{12}, and magnesium:** These key nutrients are particularly important for energy (see Chapter 4 for more on testing). A well-tolerated iron supplement is Niferex (available only by prescription). Try B_{12} injections or supplements (500–1,000 micrograms [mcg] a day). Take 400–800 mg of elemental magnesium per day (citrate, taurate, or glycinate).

- **DHEA, testosterone:** Some cases of chronic fatigue may be related to low levels of DHEA or testosterone (see Chapter 4 for testing information). By supplementing with natural hormones, energy often returns. See a physician familiar with bio-identical hormone replacement (see Resources for Patients for more on natural HRT).

- **Food allergies:** While many conventional physicians and allergists reject the notion that food allergies cause CFS, the wrong foods *can* cause exhaustion and lethargy. In particular, gluten grains (like wheat, rye, barley and oats), dairy, and yeast products lead the hit parade of fatigue suspects. Blood tests, such as the IgG RAST and the anti-gliadin antibody test, can pinpoint food allergies (see Chapter 4). Eliminating culprit foods often boosts energy.

- **Mercury, lead, chemical exposure:** Environmental toxins can poison metabolic pathways that are responsible for energy production. The nervous system is particularly vulnerable to these agents. Early symptoms of toxin overload include fatigue and malaise. Cleaning up your diet and using supplements to enhance detoxification can reduce toxic burden and restore energy (see Chapter 4).

- **Intestinal toxicity:** Sometimes toxins come from within. Poor diet and excess use of antibiotics and acid-blockers can result in dysbiosis (abnormal intestinal fermentation). In turn, overgrowth of harmful yeast and bacterial species results in production of harmful endotoxins. Better diet and probiotics (good bacteria in yogurt or supplements) can help combat this intestinal toxicity. Also consider antifungal medications, like nystatin, Diflucan, or Sporanox; or antifungal herbs (oregano, olive leaf, black walnut, pau d'arco). Read *The Yeast Connection,* by William Crook, M.D.

- **Natural adrenal support:** The adrenal glands produce several hormones and are the body's bulwark against stress. Occasionally the adrenals burn out and stop responding (see Chapter 4 for testing information). Natural adrenal support includes taking herbal remedies, such as licorice, ginseng, ashwaganda (used in traditional Indian medicine) and rosavin (from the *Rhodiola rosea* plant).

Anxiety Disorders

It's not clear whether poor diet and lifestyle are somehow contributing to the wave of anxiety, or if it's something about our frenetic, disconnected lifestyle. But anxiety disorders are a major reason people consult holistic doctors. Part of the reason is that medication alone doesn't always work against phobias, panic disorders, and generalized anxiety. Or it offers only stop-gap relief. Thankfully, there are a variety of non-drug options that can buttress mainstream medications and good therapy:

- **Cognitive behavioral therapies (CBT):** While not formally an alternative therapy, CBT is nonetheless a non-pharmacological approach to anxiety

CHANGING DIRECTIONS MIDSTREAM: BACKING OFF CONVENTIONAL TREATMENTS

When Terry Mallin began feeling tired, achy, and nauseated a few months ago, he assumed he had the flu. But when the symptoms persisted, he finally went to his doctor. After ruling out several conditions, his doctor concluded that his symptoms indicated he had chronic fatigue syndrome.

He immediately put Terry on several prescription medications, including a painkiller for the achy muscles, a selective serotonin re-uptake inhibitor (SSRI) to help him sleep and boost his mood, and an antispasmodic drug to relieve his abdominal discomfort. The drugs worked for awhile, but also produced increasingly severe side effects, including anxiety, agitation, drowsiness, and greater abdominal pain. Even after altering dosages and trying new prescriptions the side effects continued.

Terry finally did some research and concluded that throwing conventional drugs at his problem probably wasn't the answer. He also began to suspect that something else might be at the root of his condition. His doctor, though, was harder to convince.

Terry: Dr. Singer, I'm beginning to wonder if this might be a case of hypothyroidism or something like food allergies instead of chronic fatigue. Does it make sense to run more tests and think about other treatments?

disorders. The emphasis of this "talk therapy" is not to recount traumatic episodes or solve a patient's life dilemmas; rather it involves reframing patients' experience of anxiety and teaches them practical techniques for breaking the vicious cycle of maladaptive thoughts and physiological reactions. Research shows that CBT can change levels of neurotransmitters in the brain, even without medication.

• **Yoga:** The key to yoga's calming effect is proper breathing. Traditional yoga—but not Westernized incarnations like "yogaerobics"—emphasizes calm, relaxed breathing that centers on the diaphragm. Breath awareness is vital to avoiding hyperventilation, which unleashes stress hormones. Check your local "Y" or hospital for yoga classes near you.

• **Blood sugar:** Stress can result from external circumstances, or it can arise from internal causes. A prime trigger for the release of stress hormones is low blood sugar, often the result of a diet too rich in sugar and refined carbohydrates (see Chapter 9 for more on blood sugar and brain function).

Dr. Singer: I really think we ought to keep on with the medications I prescribed. Sometimes, they take awhile to work. We can continue to play around with the dosages if you're still having side effects.

Terry: I appreciate what you're saying, but I'd really like to look at other possible causes and maybe try a new diet or nutritional therapies. I have a lot of documentation here to back me up, if you want to see it.

Dr. Singer: Terry, I know the side effects are annoying, but I don't think we should mess around with anything new right now. Of course, I can't force you.

Terry: Dr. Singer, I'm sorry, but my gut just tells me to go in this other direction—at least for a while. If you'll work with me, I promise to go back on the meds if I don't get relief.

Dr. Singer: Okay, but I'll want to monitor you throughout. Let's give it a shot.

After several tests, Dr. Singer determined that Terry's thyroid function was borderline and agreed to put him on a natural thyroid extract. Tests also confirmed that Terry had sensitivity to wheat and dairy products. After eliminating them from his diet and supplementing with amino acids, magnesium, iron, and other vitamins, Terry's energy gradually returned.

- **Neurotransmitters:** The body responds to overproduction of adrenaline (resulting from anxiety) by producing "feel-good" neurotransmitters, like serotonin. Hence the popular use of serotonin-enhancing antidepressants (SSRIs, or selective serotonin reuptake inhibitors) to treat anxiety disorders. However, before turning to these powerful drugs, consider supplementing with neurotransmitter building blocks, like L-tyrosine and 5-HTP, which help here as they do in chronic fatigue (see above).

- **Magnesium:** Overproduction of adrenaline also prompts excessive magnesium loss from the kidneys. Animal experiments show that livestock subject to the stress of crowding and transport survive better if given magnesium. Take 400–800 mg of elemental magnesium per day (citrate, taurate, or glycinate).

- **Inositol, P5P:** These B vitamins exert a calming effect. Inositol helps relieve anxiety at doses of 12–15 grams a day (or 1 teaspoon of powder dissolved in cold water three times daily). Take 50–100 mg of P5P (pyridoxal-5-phosphate)—an activated form of vitamin B_6—two or three times daily.

- **Progesterone:** When women reach thirty-five or forty, or when they're stressed out, an imbalance often develops between the hormones progesterone and estrogen: progesterone plummets, and estrogen—augmented by weight gain and environmental xenoestrogens from pollutants—soars. The problem of "estrogen dominance" is further magnified by inefficient liver function. Since estrogen is linked to mood swings, the result can be anxiety. Interestingly, progesterone (the hormone of pregnancy) has the opposite effect. Indeed, many pregnant women report a calm that leads them to consider remaining "barefoot and pregnant" for as long as possible. Daily topical application of natural progesterone (available as Femgest or Progest cream) seems to alleviate hormonal stress and tension. Suggested dosage: Apply 1 tablespoon to skin daily (stop during menstruation).

Depression and Mood Disorders

Sometimes it's hard to tell the difference between anxiety and depression. As mentioned before, the same drugs are frequently used to treat both. Depression may also rear its head in many physical ailments, like CFS and fibromyalgia. Hence, some of the same treatment strategies apply to all these ailments.

While I'm no Tom Cruise, I agree that medication is often prescribed too quickly when the cause of depression remains unexplored. Fortunately, natural therapies abound to either bolster psychiatric drugs or replace them altogether.

- **Essential fatty acids:** Research by Harvard psychiatrist Andrew Stoll shows that omega-3 fatty acids in fish oil, especially EPA (eicosapentaenoic acid), play a role in mood elevation and stabilization. Even patients with suicidal depression were helped in one study (but don't try this nutritional therapy alone in lieu of psychiatric care!). Dosage is three to six 1,000-mg capsules of EPA/DHA daily. Remember, too, that persistence pays off: the best results are obtained after supplementing for three or four months, sometimes up to a year.

• **Neurotransmitters:** Ditto for supplementing with amino acids that support neurotransmitter function (see above under CFS and anxiety).

• **Insulin resistance:** Recent studies show a surprising connection between type 2 diabetes (whose key feature is insulin resistance) and depression. See Chapter 6 for more on insulin resistance. However, researchers still don't fully understand the link. Does depression lead to carbohydrate craving and sedentary habits? Or is the reverse true: insulin resistance somehow activates the lethargy and unstable moods of depression? Whatever the mechanism, I can verify that most of my insulin-resistant patients report better mood and energy when they exercise, lose weight, eat the Salad and Salmon diet (see Resources for Patients), and take supplements, like chromium and alpha-lipoic acid, which improve insulin response.

• **Exercise:** In addition to its blood-sugar stabilizing effects, exercise is also a natural endorphin-enhancer. Endorphins are neurotransmitters that relieve stress and boost mood. Both aerobic activities (like running, swimming, and cycling), as well as weight training, have this effect. Get your daily exercise "fix" to heighten mood and help stave off less healthy food cravings.

• **SAM-e:** S-adenosylmethionine is an amino acid with remarkable mood-enhancing powers. Popularized in the United States by Columbia University psychiatrist Richard Brown in his book *Stop Depression Now,* SAM-e has been shown to safely enhance the benefits of most antidepressants, or it can be taken alone. I recommend 400–600 mg twice daily.

• **St. John's wort:** While controversy rages after a series of negative studies showed that St. John's wort isn't effective even in mild-to-moderate depression, I still think it can work for selected patients. The problem is that it interacts with many medications, rendering them less potent. Therefore, I recommend it only for patients not taking prescription drugs. Take 300 mg of the standardized extract three times daily. Note: Some people taking St. John's wort report extreme sensitivity to sunlight, so avoid heavy sun exposure.

• **DHEA, testosterone:** Several studies suggest that DHEA and testosterone can boost mood in both men and women who suffer from aging-associated depression. Supplementing with these hormones may be especially effective in women who've had their ovaries surgically removed—not just sex drive but overall well-being improves. Other studies show that older men are less "grumpy" when DHEA and testosterone are restored to youthful levels. See a physician familiar with bio-identical hormone replacement.

• **Thyroid:** As with CFS, hidden hypothyroidism may also play a role in depression. Interestingly, psychiatrists, like holistic physicians, are the only doctors who sometimes urge their patients to "take a little thyroid." That's because many antidepressant drugs are actually strengthened by prescription thyroid. Speak to your doctor about taking a natural thyroid extract.

• **Folic acid:** Also tell your doctor about little-known studies showing that high doses of folic acid (1–5 grams per day) can significantly enhance the therapeutic effects of most antidepressants, including fluoxetine (Prozac) and other SSRIs.[3,4]

Andropause

Some people think andropause was invented solely to promote hormone interventions for self-indulgent baby-boomer men. But I disagree. While not as clearly defined as female menopause, andropause is real. It can occur abruptly or very gradually—as early as thirty-five or as late as the mid-seventies. The good news is that many interventions exist to help men through this period of intense physiologic change.

• **Testosterone, DHEA:** For andropause, nothing works like "the real thing": bio-identical hormone replacement via topical creams, gels, capsules, sublingual lozenges, patches, or injections. But just as women who receive HRT must undergo frequent surveillance to rule out breast or uterine cancer, so men must also be carefully monitored for prostate and other cancers. The Life Extension Foundation offers a factual website on natural hormone replacement for men. www.lef.org/protocols/prtcl-130.shtml.

• **Saw palmetto:** Of all herbal therapies, saw palmetto extract for prevention and reversal of benign prostatic hypertrophy (BPH), or enlarged prostate, is most well documented. Take 320 mg daily of standardized saw palmetto extract (it should contain 85 to 95 percent fatty acids and sterols—the main ingredients).

• **Insulin resistance:** During andropause, falling DHEA and testosterone levels often conspire with insulin resistance to cause debilitation and physical decline. It's a vicious cycle: fatigue and lack of initiative from declining androgens promote weight gain, body fat accumulation, and lower muscle mass. As fat continues to accumulate, insulin levels soar. In turn, rising levels of sex hormone–binding globulin (SHBG) tie up even more circulating androgens.

The result? Middle-aged men often find themselves increasingly fatigued, fat, and emasculated. Reversing this downward spiral requires a change in diet (see Chapter 6 for nutritional strategies to combat insulin resistance).

• **Strength training:** Cardio workouts may appeal to aging boomer men trying to recapture past athletic glory, but bodybuilding is important, too. In fact, strength training counters insulin resistance, fortifies testosterone levels naturally, and helps slow sarcopenia, muscle loss that otherwise proceeds at a rate of 10 percent per decade. Check with your doctor before starting, and try getting some tips from a certified personal trainer to avoid injuries and get the most out of your workout (see Chapter 6 for more on strength training).

Menopause

I object to calling menopause a disorder; it's actually a natural change not unlike puberty. Some women transit gracefully through the end of their periods with scarcely a complaint while others have devastating symptoms. Still others find it harder to maintain optimal body proportions and begin to age rapidly. I consider menopause an opportunity to take stock of your health assets and liabilities, and begin a program of corrective action, preferably via natural means.

• **Syndrome W:** My colleague Harriette R. Mogul, M.D., introduced the concept of Syndrome W—a collection of health problems that begin around menopause. These include declining sex hormones, worsening insulin resistance with weight gain, high cholesterol, high blood pressure, and eventually diabetes. Subtle thyroid problems may also develop, causing more weight gain. In addition, the stress of this mid-life transition bathes the body in cortisol, a steroid hormone which also fosters fat accumulation. To prevent this kind of debilitation, Syndrome W must be addressed on all fronts, including eating a low-carb diet and exercising. Read Dr. Mogul's book *Syndrome W: A Woman's Guide to Reversing Mid-Life Weight Gain.*

• **Natural alternatives to HRT:** CAM remedies abound for hot flashes and other menopausal discomforts. One of the most popular is black cohosh—the leading herbal therapy for hot flashes in Europe. Though study results are mixed, I find it works about 40 percent of the time (but only on hot flashes and not mood swings or vaginal dryness). Some experts worry about harmful effects from plant estrogens that may pose a danger to breasts and uterus. But most studies suggest this isn't the case—black cohosh seems to work by acting on the pituitary. My favorite product is Remifemin (containing the type of black cohosh researched in Germany). Take one to two capsules twice daily.

• **Bio-identical HRT:** Hormone therapy took a major hit after the results of the Women's Health Initiative (see Chapter 6). But I still think there's a place for balanced hormone replacement, particularly for women with devastating menopausal symptoms. I recommend natural hormones that replicate what women make before menopause, including estriol, estradiol, progesterone, DHEA, and testosterone. There's no "one-size-fits-all" approach to dosage or delivery. Patches, creams, pills, and sublingual lozenges all have advantages with various dosages and combinations. Consult a practitioner familiar with prescribing natural hormones (check out the American College for Advancement in Medicine for possible providers: www.acam.org).

• **Osteoporosis prevention:** Many women confront this bone-thinning condition at midlife. The same goes for its precursor, osteopenia (if ever there was a "disease that isn't a disease" this natural process of bone aging would be it). Getting a vitamin D check is essential at menopause. Other nutrients that enhance the benefits of calcium for bone retention include magnesium, boron, vitamin K, the mineral silica, the amino acid L-lysine, the plant-derived compound ipriflavone, phytoestrogens from soy, and the mineral strontium citrate. (See Resources for Patients for more on my product Osteosupport.)

Sexual Dysfunction

Let's get one thing straight—I don't believe in "natural" aphrodisiacs. Millions are spent yearly on "sexual cocktails" for men and women with exotic sounding names like maca, muira puama, and *Tribulus terrestris.* Yet all are without real scientific proof. Granted, some may provide a placebo benefit, but it's still probably cheaper to buy a rabbit's foot!

More impressive, but with only slightly more proof, are claims that high doses of L-arginine have a Viagra-like effect (both stimulate nitric oxide production); that ginkgo biloba reverses sexual problems in those on antidepressants; and that ginseng and rhodiola raise testosterone, DHEA, and growth hormones. However, before you stock up on questionable herbal remedies or pick up a Viagra prescription, consider the following strategies:

• **Bio-identical HRT:** Suzanne Somers created a sensation with her bestselling book *The Sexy Years,* suggesting that balanced supplementation with natural hormones can promote sexual functioning well past menopause. In fact, studies show that DHEA levels correspond reasonably well with a woman's reported sexual desire and response. However, trials of testosterone supplementation have met with mixed reviews. The one exception is women who've had their ovaries removed as part of a "total hysterectomy." Testosterone replacement is necessary not just to restore sex drive, but also to stabilize mood.

• **Check your medicine cabinet:** Numerous medications can interfere with sex drive, especially blood pressure drugs and antidepressants. This isn't necessarily an alternative medicine intervention, but by using natural means like diet, exercise, and the non-drug options outlined in this book, you may find you don't need all these medications that kill sex drive and impair performance.

• **Get healthy:** As a teaser on my radio show, I announced one weekend that I was going to reveal the natural secret to great sex—at a cost of only pennies a day! Listeners probably sat riveted to their radios waiting for me to describe the latest vitamin or herbal panacea. What they got instead was the lowdown on health and fitness—sorry about that! The truth is a good diet and exercise pays dividends in the bedroom. Indeed, studies show that sedentary people who lose weight and boost fitness report more and better sex.

• **Neurotransmitters:** Research indicates that the brain chemical dopamine boosts sex drive and response. Interestingly, new dopamine-raising drugs used to treat restless leg syndrome sometimes cause an inadvertent spike in sex drive (even prompting some disgruntled patients and their partners to file class-action lawsuits against the drug manufacturers!) Of course, there are gentler natural ways to support dopamine production in the body using natural amino acid precursors like L-tyrosine. Be sure to work with a nutritional practitioner experienced in measuring and balancing neurotransmitters.

Fibromyalgia

Fibromyalgia is characterized by achy body, fatigue, depression, poor sleep, and sometimes gastrointestinal symptoms. Patients also exhibit pairs of tender points on their shoulders, arms, legs and torso, which are sensitive to pressure. A great book on fibromyalgia is *From Fatigued to Fantastic!*, by Jacob Teitelbaum, M.D.

Because fibromyalgia and CFS sufferers share common symptoms, I treat FMS (fibromyalgia syndrome) similarly to CFS (see above)—but with a few added considerations:

• **Vitamin D:** One of the best-kept secrets in nutrition is that some patients suffering from mysterious muscle pains are low in vitamin D. In fact, research shows that dark-skinned individuals with vague aches and pains are often low in D (darker skin requires more time in the sun to make it). When D is restored, the majority report that their aches and pains disappear! Have your doctor test your vitamin D levels. If low, take 1,000–4,000 international units (IU) of natural vitamin D3 (but make sure to keep track of your D levels so you don't overshoot the mark!). Also, try to get controlled time in the sun (fifteen to forty-five minutes per day).

• **Myers Cocktail:** A mainstay of holistic physicians, the Myers Cocktail is an intravenous injection rich in magnesium, B vitamins, and vitamin C. The late John Myers, M.D., the Baltimore physician who invented it, attracted a large clientele of fibromyalgia patients in the 1970s and 1980s until his retirement. The Myers Cocktail treatment is currently being studied at Yale University by David Katz, M.D., under a research grant from the National Center for Complementary and Alternative Medicine (NCCAM). For a list of practitioners trained to administer the Myers Cocktail, visit the American College for Advancement in Medicine: www.acam.org.

• **Food allergy:** As we saw in Chapter 8, food intolerance can be a source of arthritis and other kinds of pain. The mechanism is not classic food allergy, but rather a ramping up of cytokine production, which is akin to what happens when you get the flu. Cytokines are chemical messengers that help regulate the immune system and spring into action at the first sign of foreign invaders. When someone has sensitivity to certain foods, such as wheat, milk, sugar, soy, peanuts, corn or eggs, the immune system mistakes these menu items for viral or bacterial intruders. The resulting excess cytokine production can cause achiness, fever, and extreme fatigue. To determine whether your fibromyalgia symptoms are really food sensitivity, ask your doctor for an IgG RAST test (see Chapter 4), or eliminate suspect foods.

• **Neurotransmitters:** As in CFS, balancing neurotransmitters can be helpful in FMS, as well. Research suggests that pain might not originate in the muscles, but instead arises from neurotransmitter dysfunction in the brain. Improving neurotransmitter balance not only reduces pain but also facilitates sleep—immensely beneficial to FMS sufferers.

• **Bio-identical HRT:** Many men who suffer from fibromyalgia turn out to have low testosterone and DHEA. The vast majority of FMS patients are women, but it stands to reason that these androgens may provide protection against their aches and pains, as well. In fact, some but not all sufferers of FMS feel better after treatment with bio-identical hormones.

• **Ribose:** One of the newer therapies on the FMS scene, ribose (a carbohydrate found naturally in cells) acts to energize the muscles, helping them perform more efficiently. Borrowed from bodybuilding, the theory is that ribose is a precursor to ATP (adenosine triphosphate), an energy compound made in muscles. Suggested dosage: 1 teaspoon (5 mg) of ribose powder three times daily in water.

Adult ADD

This is one of those vogue diagnoses, currently all the rage. Drug company websites abound, inviting visitors to take a "self-test" for adult ADD (attention-deficit disorder). If you are "easily bored," "fidget a lot," or have "inconsistent work performance," you could be among the estimated millions of adult ADD sufferers. And if so, there are a slew of new psychiatric drugs—field-tested on kids—to help.

But is it really ADD or the fast-paced demands of our multi-tasking society? Whatever the cause, there are clearly many adults who are distracted, underperforming, and subject to "brain-fog." However, before you begin popping powerful attention-focusing drugs like Ritalin or Adderall, first consider the following strategies:

- **Blood sugar:** Hypoglycemic reactions are a big culprit in both adult and childhood ADD. While doctors acknowledge that diabetics on insulin can have brain-addling episodes of low blood sugar, most believe ordinary folks are exempt. Ask your doctor for a glucose tolerance test (see Chapter 4), and consider yourself hypoglycemic if you feel increasingly restless and lack focus as your blood sugar plummets after three or four hours. Then begin a low-glycemic diet with slower-acting carbohydrates (like whole grains) that don't raise blood sugar quickly and plenty of protein to anchor your blood sugar. See www.glycemicindex.com.

- **Food allergy:** Food reactions go beyond just itching, sniffling, and wheezing: foods like wheat and dairy can also trigger a brain-muddling effect in sensitive individuals. The fog lifts when these foods are removed. Ask your doctor for an IgG RAST test, or try an elimination diet.

- **Neurotransmitters:** Concentration is a function of having optimal brain levels of neurotransmitters. Just as balancing neurotransmitters often helps depression and anxiety, it can also sometimes reverse brain fog. Of special interest in ADD is L-theanine, a non-caffeine compound found in tea. Research shows that L-theanine promotes alpha-wave activity in the brain (as does meditation), which is linked to relaxed focus. Drink a cup or two of black or green tea daily. Or take one or two L-theanine capsules two or three times daily.

- **Thyroid:** Difficulty concentrating and lack of focus are sometimes signs of hypothyroidism. Even where thyroid tests are borderline or low normal, a targeted dose of natural thyroid medication, like Armour Thyroid or Euthroid, can restore mental sharpness as well as amphetamine-like ADD drugs.

- **Get a sleep checkup:** Unbeknownst to many ADD sufferers, daytime symptoms may be the result of sleep deprivation. Sometimes it's deliberate (inadequate time budgeted for sleep) or a problem of insomnia. Occasionally, the culprit is sleep apnea—sufferers log normal hours in bed, but their sleep is compromised by episodes of breathlessness. A sleep study at a sleep laboratory can cinch the diagnosis of sleep apnea and help with treatment.

- **Iron deficiency** often clouds thinking. In fact, women and girls with low iron (the result of monthly blood loss during their periods or from multiple childbirths) can literally lose up to 10 to 20 IQ points! People on vegetarian diets are also at greater risk. Ask your doctor for a ferritin test (see Chapter 4). Even if you're not overtly anemic or iron-deficient by conventional criteria, your ferritin score shouldn't be lower than 40 or 50 for optimal mental focus.

Reflux Disease (GERD)

Gastroesophageal reflux disease is a classic example of how bothersome but minor symptoms, like heartburn and indigestion, often become elevated to "disease" status. Behind GERD's recent rise to prominence are a slew of new ultra-powerful acid blockers, some of which are now even available over the counter. But in my experience these potent drugs are seldom necessary when natural approaches are used.

- **Weight loss:** Being overweight increases the risk of GERD by 50 percent. While normal-weight people with GERD abound, they are the exception to the rule. Abdominal fat puts pressure on the stomach and forces its contents back up into the esophagus, resulting in distressing symptoms and discomfort.

- **Food intolerance:** Some foods cause GERD, either because they tend to "float" like lighter-than-water fat or bubbly soda, or because they relax the pyloric sphincter, a valve that keeps food in the stomach. Foods that do the latter include chocolate and peppermint. In addition, there are caustic foods—like coffee, alcohol, and spicy dishes—that simply irritate. Many people also have their own individual patterns of food intolerance: for some it may be wheat, for others dairy, and still others may not tolerate raw cruciferous vegetables. Finally, some individuals are highly sensitive to food additives; one of the most persistent in GERD is MSG (monosodium glutamate). Unfortunately, uncovering it in your diet can be tricky since MSG goes by many pseudonyms. Ask your doctor about blood tests, such as the IgG RAST and the anti-gliadin antibody test, to pinpoint food allergies (see Chapter 4).

- **Fermentation:** During Prohibition when moonshine was covertly fermented in the Ozarks and Appalachia, occasionally you'd hear of disastrous explosions—the high-pressure contents of some hidden still would just erupt volcanically. Some cases of GERD result from a similar process of fermentation (only it happens in the upper gastrointestinal tract). Remember Ben? All it takes is starch in the presence of sugar and yeast—picture your typical American breakfast of cereal, milk, and orange juice, and voilà, you have a burbling, fermenting mix just waiting to explode. A diet switch to high-protein foods and low-starch vegetables, along with probiotics and antifungal medications

(Nystatin, Diflucan, or Sporanox) or antifungal herbs (oregano, olive leaf, black walnut, pau d'arco), often corrects the problem.

• **DGL, aloe:** Deglycyrrhizinated licorice, or DGL, packs the anti-inflammatory punch of licorice without its blood-pressure-raising and potassium-depleting side effects. Dissolve six to twelve lozenges in your mouth throughout the day (away from meals) to coat your esophagus with healing DGL. An additional treatment (although less palatable for some) is fresh aloe extract (I prefer the thick gel to the juice). Take $\frac{1}{4}$ cup (2 ounces), three or four times daily, on an empty stomach.

• **Stress reduction, meditation:** Stress also fosters GERD: either by directly interfering with normal gastric emptying, literally causing food to "stick in your craw," or by indirectly promoting fast and indiscriminate eating. See Resources for Patients for more on stress reduction and meditation techniques.

Irritable Bowel Syndrome (IBS)

Once a "waste-basket" diagnosis that doctors tossed out when they couldn't pinpoint a clear-cut cause of belly pain, IBS has since risen to the level of "real" ailment. Many drugs are now available that target the complex intestinal nerve network controlling cramping and irregularity. Yet they don't seem to work for everyone. I've long been a proponent of natural strategies for troubleshooting IBS and even wrote a book about it in 1988, called *Seven Weeks to a Settled Stomach*. Over the years, I've seen many sufferers achieve substantial relief with the following approaches:

• **Food intolerance:** A recent study showed that when culprit foods are identified via an IgG RAST allergy test and eliminated, IBS symptoms often disappear.[5] Additionally, many patients have individual intolerances to other foods, such as lactose (milk sugar), fructose and/or sorbitol (fruit sugars) and certain difficult-to-digest fibers or starches (brussel's sprouts or granola, for example). See Chapter 4 for more on food allergy testing.

• **Gluten intolerance:** It's now recognized that up to 1 to 2 percent of Americans may have celiac disease, a severe intolerance to wheat, barley, rye and other grains, but most remain undiagnosed. In fact, a considerable number of IBS sufferers may fall into this category or have a gluten intolerance that does not quite meet the formal criteria of celiac disease (confirmed by intestinal biopsy). The anti-gliadin antibody test can pinpoint patients who might benefit from eliminating dietary gluten (see Chapter 4).

• **Probiotics:** As discussed above under GERD, overgrowth of abnormal bacteria and yeast in the intestinal tract promotes bloating and gas. Replacing them with normal intestinal bacteria (found in probiotic-containing yogurt or supplements) often eliminates IBS symptoms.

• **Candida, parasites:** Other unwelcome inhabitants in the intestinal tract also cause distress. In addition to medication, which your doctor can prescribe, natural antimicrobial herbs like oregano, olive leaf, black walnut, pau d'arco (available in supplements) can also banish pathogens.

• **Hypnosis:** Because the brain-gut link in IBS is strong, considerable research has investigated the potential role of hypnosis in relieving IBS symptoms. The vast majority of studies are positive. Subjects are trained to induce a relaxed state and then are asked to visualize waves of healing energy or soothing color flowing to their gut. Ask your doctor for the name of a qualified hypnotherapist or check with the National Board for Certified Clinical Hypnotherapists (see Resources for Patients).

• **Peppermint oil:** Certain herbs are said to have carminative, or anti-spasmodic, effects. Chief among them are peppermint and spearmint. Try drinking mint tea, or better yet, take *enteric-coated* peppermint oil capsules, which are designed to time-release in the lower intestine where they do their job on cramps. Take two capsules four times daily between meals and at bedtime.

Throughout this chapter, we've seen that many seemingly severe health problems are actually the result of nutritional deficiencies, poor lifestyle, or underlying health issues that can be treated holistically with gentler CAM therapies. Of course, some health conditions require the heavy artillery of mainstream medicine. But even these treatments can usually be complemented with natural therapies that minimize side effects and enhance effectiveness. This includes surgery, as we'll see in the next chapter,

Preparing for
Surgery and Recovery

Surgeons must be very careful when they take the knife!
Underneath their fine incisions, stirs the culprit—Life!
—Emily Dickinson

Back in medical school, I went through a series of "clerkships"—the practical part of medical training where students leave the classroom to walk the hospital halls and act like junior doctors. There was psychiatry, where I discovered an extraordinary ability to discuss delusions with the mentally ill. There was ob-gyn where I birthed babies; pediatrics where I ministered to sick kids; and internal medicine, my chosen field, where I toiled alongside young doctors in an inner-city hospital ward. And then there was surgery.

Unexpectedly, I showed a certain knack in the surgery suite that impressed the house staff and attending surgeons. I didn't get to do much actual cutting, but my stitching was passable, and I could hold retractors with the best of them. After receiving an "Honors" grade, I was confronted with a dilemma: could I achieve my career goal of bringing innovation to medicine within the high-tech discipline of surgery?

The answer, to my surprise, was a definite "maybe." I learned that surgeons care a lot about nutrition, maybe more so than their internal-medicine colleagues. Surgeons know that malnourished patients make them look bad, and even the deftest surgeon can be stymied by post-operative complications resulting from poor wound healing, shock, and suppressed immunity that leads to infections. A surgeon is only as good as his or her stats, and unnecessary deaths and days spent languishing in the intensive-care unit (ICU) reflect poorly on success rates.

Therefore, many surgeons use nutritional support aggressively before and immediately after surgery to optimize results. Indeed, a rich, evidence-based scientific literature has emerged around the role that several perioperative nutrients play in optimizing recovery (from hospitalization to discharge). Some may eventually become regular therapeutic adjuncts to surgery.

We'll cover the most promising of these therapies in this chapter. You'll want to discuss them with your surgeon. We'll also look at the idea of "pre-hab"—steps you can take before surgery to ensure the best healing and recovery possible.

UNNECESSARY SURGERY

Long before you begin preparing for surgery, be sure that it's your only option. Statistics suggest that millions of unnecessary surgeries are performed each year. The American College of Surgeons recommends asking these questions before opting for an operation:

- What are the indications for this procedure?
- What, if any, alternative forms of treatment are available?
- What will be the likely result if you don't have the operation?
- What are the risks?
- How is the operation expected to improve your health or quality of life?
- Are there likely to be residual effects from the operation?

If, after discussing these questions, you feel that surgery is your best option, it's fine to forgo a second opinion. However, if you're having doubts, you may want to consult someone else. Check out the American College of Surgeon's guide to seeking a surgical second opinion (www.facs.org/public_info/operation/consult.html). See "The Art of the Deal" on page 195 for tips on negotiating how much your surgeon can cut during a procedure.

CRUEL PARADOX

As you begin preparing your body and mind for surgery, don't be surprised if you meet some resistance. Surgeons may increasingly rely on pre- and post-op nutritional support, but there's one rub: hospitals continue to *actively dissuade* patients from using nutrition to improve their odds of successful surgery.

Witness the rise of glitzy MacDonalds, Burger Kings, and KFCs in place of stodgy hospital cafeterias. To paraphrase an old saying, the true art of the surgeon lies in preventing surgery. By condoning junk food and other poor health habits, hospitals are, at best, missing the boat, and at worst, are in serious breech of their medical responsibility.

Even worse, many hospitals now deliberately undercut patients' efforts to optimize nutritional support before and after surgery because they fear that use of herbs and supplements might lead to potential complications and/or drug-nutrient interactions.

THE ART OF THE DEAL: NEGOTIATING HOW MUCH TO CUT

Forty-nine-year-old Marissa Morton was diagnosed with uterine fibroids and a small ovarian cyst a year ago. After a period of "watchful waiting," her doctor recently informed her that her fibroids were growing significantly (her uterus had swelled to the size of a four-month pregnancy) and recommended a hysterectomy to stop profuse bleeding during her periods. He also suggested removing her ovaries at the same time, even though the cyst wasn't causing problems or growing ("just to be safe").

At first Marissa agreed, but after doing a web search she began to wonder whether an ovariectomy was really necessary or advisable. Ovaries are vital for hormone balance, even after menopause (in fact, women who immediately go on HRT are still much more prone to problems of aging, including heart disease, as well as fatigue and depression). Here she negotiates with her surgeon about what and how much to cut.

Marissa: From what you've said in the past, I'm really not sure I need my ovaries out.

Dr. Chambers: Look, you've completed your family. You don't need ovaries anymore. I only suggested removing them because we'll already be in there—we'll just clean things up a bit and reduce your risk of cancer.

Marissa: But you told me not to worry about ovarian cancer because I don't have a family history or other risk factors. I'm just not sure I'm ready for immediate menopause, if it isn't necessary.

Dr. Chambers: Actually it's pretty standard for someone your age with cysts to get their ovaries removed. But I guess we could just remove the cyst.

Marissa: But didn't you say that most cysts eventually disappear on their own, especially after menopause. Do we even have to go that far since the cyst is small and looks benign?

Dr. Chambers: Well, I suppose not . . . okay, here's what we'll do. Let me take a closer look for anything suspicious when I'm in there. If something looks funny, I'd like to remove the cyst, but not your ovaries. We'll test it for cancer and go from there. If it looks okay, I'll leave it alone, but keep monitoring it. How does that sound?

Marissa: It's a deal.

Why the Commotion?

Hospitals aren't wrong to worry about potential interactions. Complications can happen, though they usually involve only a handful of herbs and supplements. Unfortunately, fears are fanned because many patients don't share which supplements they're taking with surgeons. In one study of patients receiving general medical care (not just surgery), half failed to disclose their use of herbal medicines unless directly asked—perhaps out of fear that their doctor would disapprove.[1] Other studies show that patients also commonly fail to report their use of over-the-counter (OTC) medications that may need to be halted before surgery, like aspirin.

To me the message isn't that patients should avoid *all* herbal and OTC medications a week before surgery (a common practice at many hospitals). I think blanket restrictions are overkill and deprive patients of the real and tangible benefits of properly administered nutritional support. What's really needed is more communication between doctors and patients. That means patients should speak up and doctors should ask for a detailed history of supplements long before patients are wheeled into the OR.[2]

The following are four types of potential drug-nutrient interactions that surgeons and anesthesiologists watch out for, as well as a few supplements and herbs that can cause them. Some, you might want to halt. Others, though, may actually be helpful before and after surgery. Educate yourself and talk to your surgeon.

Hemostasis (Coagulation and Clotting)

Like aspirin and other blood thinners, such as Coumadin, certain herbs and vitamins also have blood-thinning effects. Depending on the type of surgery you're having, this may lead to excessive bleeding. You may want to err on the side of caution and halt most of these anticoagulants five to seven days prior to surgery.

However, before you swear them off altogether, remember that an anticoagulant effect can be beneficial during some lengthy surgeries where patients are at risk for blood clots because they're immobilized for so long. Additionally, some supplements, like fish oil and vitamin E, only act as blood thinners when taken at higher doses, but may offer inherent healing powers when used at lower doses. Be sure to discuss using the following supplements well before your operation:

- **Garlic:** Garlic supplements have a platelet-inhibiting effect, and at least one report has shown that garlic pills may promote increased bleeding into the eyeball after delicate cataract surgery.

- **Ginger:** No actual research confirms that the potential blood-thinning properties of ginger boost surgery risk. In fact, its use has been advocated to forestall post-procedure nausea (see "Revisiting Controversies" on page 208). Nevertheless, you may want to consider curtailing pre-op use as a precaution.

• **Ginkgo biloba:** Because this herb inhibits the formation of clots, it probably shouldn't be taken before surgery. However, the risk may turn out to be more theoretical than real: a soon-to-be-published study failed to show any increase in bleeding, either alone or in combination with aspirin.

• **Feverfew:** Likewise for this anti-migraine herb, often cited as a no-no prior to surgery.

• **Chinese herbs:** Several Chinese herbs, including dong quai (*Angelica sinensis*) and dan shen (red sage), come under the general category of "blood movers" (a Chinese term) and act as mild anticoagulants. Many are ingredients in many mixed herbal formulas and may go by different names. Best bet: Stop taking all Chinese herbs before surgery.

• **Vitamin E:** While vitamin E is known to be a blood thinner at high doses, most studies suggest that these effects don't emerge if you take less than 400 international units (IU) a day. Additionally, E plays a key role in preventing immune suppression and free-radical damage, as well as in promoting wound healing. We'll discuss the potential benefits of taking vitamin E for surgery in greater detail below.

• **Fish oil:** We'll also look at omega-3 oils, which are blood thinners but may offer distinct benefits for surgical patients at lower doses, as well.

Sedative Effects

Sedatives, including anesthesia, are used to calm the nervous system and help patients get through surgical procedures without pain or anxiety. However, some natural sedatives, like those below, can prolong or exaggerate the impact of anesthesia—a potentially dangerous effect.

• **Kava:** Evidence suggests that residual amounts of kava in a patient's bloodstream can affect anesthesia. It's probably wise to discontinue it at least twenty-four hours before surgery.

• **Valerian:** Sleep is sometimes a problem pre-operatively, and patients may gravitate toward this natural sleep-enhancer. No studies have confirmed negative consequences when valerian is combined with anesthesia, but you should probably also halt its use twenty-four hours before surgery.

Note: Unlike the previous sedatives, research suggests that *melatonin* is a safe way to promote sleep during the perioperative period. In particular, it may be

ideal for re-adjusting patients' internal clocks and sleep cycles, often thrown off by
the disorienting effects of medication and perpetually lit hospital rooms.

Metabolism of Other Drugs

Many natural supplements can interfere with or hamper the effects of surgical
drugs, including pain and anesthetic medications. These include:

- **St. John's wort:** This popular natural antidepressant affects the body's ability to distribute, metabolize, and excrete certain medications. In fact, it often
accelerates the breakdown of certain drugs, rendering them less effective. Stop
taking a week before surgery.

- **Milk thistle:** Walk into any health-food store, and the person behind the
vitamin counter may recommend milk thistle as a way to "detoxify" your liver.
Though probably appealing to surgical candidates who dread heavy doses of
conventional drugs, milk thistle can have an unpredictable effect on drug
metabolism. Until these effects are better understood, it's best to stop taking
milk thistle a week before surgery.

Cardiovascular Effects

Cardiovascular problems such as high blood pressure and heart arrhythmias can
put you at higher risk for surgical complications, including strokes and heart
attacks. Because the following supplements may affect various cardiovascular
functions, consider avoiding them before surgery.

- **Ephedra:** Used for centuries in many cultures to treat allergies, asthma, and
upper respiratory infections, ephedra has taken a hit lately because of abuse by
dieters and recreational users. Due to its effects on blood pressure and heart
rate, it should be avoided at least twenty-four hours prior to surgery.

- **Licorice:** A valuable herb that is part of many traditional Chinese formulas,
licorice can cause problems if taken in excess because it may raise blood pressure, cause water and sodium retention, and deplete potassium. When combined with surgical drugs, its effects may be magnified. Hence it should be
discontinued a week before surgery.

PRE-HAB

If you've ever had hip or knee replacement surgery you might have stayed at a
convalescent hospital afterward. Like a halfway house from the hospital to your
home, convalescent facilities aren't just for "old fogies" anymore, but offer surgical patients of all ages convenient post-op rehab, including physical therapy and
expertly prepared meals. In fact, many seem like upscale spas, complete with fancy
gym equipment and dedicated one-on-one trainers.

Obviously, tremendous attention is given to rehab *after* surgery. But why wait to gear up for healing mode. I think it's high time we introduce the concept of pre-hab. Here are some steps you can take *before* surgery to encourage optimum recovery:

Optimize Your Weight

Consider these facts:

- Obese people are more likely to have heart disease and diabetes, putting them at significantly greater risk of surgical complications, including wound infections and cardiac events (racing heart, sudden increase in blood pressure, heart attack).

- Obese people are more likely to suffer from related vascular diseases that may also cause life-threatening complications. These include atherosclerosis (arteries clogged by fatty plaque buildup); atherothrombosis (blood clot in the artery); venous thrombosis (blood clot in the vein); and a pulmonary embolus (blood clot in a vessel of the lungs).

- Nearly half of obese people suffer from respiratory conditions, such as sleep apnea and asthma, which put them at elevated risk for respiratory complications during surgery. These include pneumonia, atelectasis (collapsed lung), and low oxygen in the blood that requires use of a ventilator or respiratory medications.

- Obesity is linked to poor immune function that diminishes the body's ability to fight against bacterial and viral invaders.

- Obese people have higher levels of oxidative stress from free radicals—which is worsened by the trauma of surgery. Free radicals destroy tissue and reduce energy production needed for cellular repair and healing.

- Overweight orthopedic patients take longer to heal after surgery because of the added load on their weight-bearing joints.

Bottom-line: Losing pounds in the pre-op period can ease rehab and get you back on your feet faster. Talk to your doctor or nutritionist about the best weight-loss strategy for you.

Get Going

A good way to lose weight is through regular exercise. I often tell patients that elective surgery is a little like military combat: Soldiers increase their combat-readiness by undertaking rigorous boot camp. You may not be ready to run obstacle courses or give the drill sergeant fifty pushups, but anything you can do to enhance heart function, lung capacity, and muscle tone prior to surgery will increase your chances of making a full recovery.

Years of research bear this out. One study of two hundred patients about to undergo open-heart surgery, for instance, found that the least physically fit (with the lowest aerobic capacity) were most likely to develop at least one surgical complication and needed a longer period of hospital rest afterward.[3] Other studies show that even mild-to-moderate exercise goes a long way toward reducing complications and enhancing post-surgical healing.

Specifically, exercise does the following:

• Reduces the risk of blood clots by keeping blood moving through vessels. (Note: *Strenuous* exercise may adversely affect the body's ability to dissolve blood clots.)

• Boosts antioxidant defenses, cutting the risk of oxidative stress from free radicals (again, heavy exercise may boost oxidative stress).

• Strengthens respiratory muscles, expands lung volume, improves the exchange of oxygen from lungs to arteries, and increases blood flow and oxygen to tissues.

• Enhances the body's immune defense against viruses and bacteria.

Relieve Stress

The months and weeks leading up to surgery can be fraught with anxiety and worry about everything from waking up during the procedure to fear of excruciating post-op pain. Unfortunately, this may slow the body's healing response and add time and pain to your recovery. One new study, for example, found that hernia patients who were worried about surgery had significantly lower levels of healing proteins and enzymes working at the wound site after the procedure.[4] The takeaway message is this: participation in stress-relieving activities beforehand can shorten hospital stays, reduce the amount of medication needed during and after surgery, cut complications, and speed recovery.

Unfortunately, few surgeons offer pre-surgery stress-relief programs (see "Practice Tips for Doctors" on page 202 for two exceptions to the rule). That's why it's important to develop your own stress-busting plan.

• **Educate yourself** about the surgery you're undergoing, the amount of pain to expect, estimated recovery times, and potential physical limitations afterward. Don't be afraid to ask questions or share your concerns about any aspect of the procedure. Research shows that most surgeons only spend about seven minutes describing upcoming operations, and a majority of patients don't feel it's adequate to alleviate fears. Make sure to read all consent and hospital forms.

According to recent studies, nearly two-thirds of patients don't read them at all. And those who do may be so scared they don't retain most of the information.

• **Work with your surgeon on a pain-control plan.** Fear of pain during and after surgery is one of patients' biggest worries. And rightly so. Studies show that many patients don't receive adequate pain relief. Ask about your pain-control options and how you can participate in managing pain yourself. Find out what pain medications will be used, how you can let the staff know if pain increases, and how pain will be relieved once you're released from the hospital.

• **Stay optimistic.** This includes learning new ways of viewing stressful events, such as reframing negative self-talk into more positive affirmations and challenging old ways of thinking that bring you down.

• **Learn relaxation techniques,** including visualization, hypnosis, imagery, and breathing exercises. If appropriate, rely on spiritual practices that have helped in the past, including prayer. You may also want to try music therapy or acupuncture (see "Revisiting Controversies" on page 208). Many of these techniques alleviate both pre- and post-op anxiety, as well as physical symptoms, including elevated blood pressure, high heart rate, release of stress hormones, muscle tension, and rapid and shallow breathing.[5]

For more on holistic approaches to pre-surgery stress, read *Preparing for Surgery: A Mind-Body Approach to Enhance Healing and Recovery,* by William W. Deardorff and John L. Reeves II.

Stop Smoking

Nicotine in any form (cigarette, patch, gum, chewing tobacco) causes your blood vessels to constrict and diminishes the amount of oxygen and nutrients that reach your tissues. In turn, surgical wounds may not adequately heal.

Oxygen delivery is particularly important when the skin is separated from underlying structures and creates a flap (especially common in cosmetic surgeries, such as facelifts, neck lifts, breast lifts, and tummy tucks). If you use nicotine, you greatly boost your chances that the skin flap will die, leaving an even uglier problem than the one you started with. In fact, the risk of complications is so high that many surgeons won't operate on patients who smoke.

Smoking also depletes vitamin C levels 40 percent quicker than in non-smokers and may boost your risk of post-op complications. One new study of three hundred cancer patients undergoing lung removal surgery found that rates of pneumonia and other lung complications were far higher in smokers (19 percent) versus non-smokers (8 percent).[6] Interestingly, the more patients smoked,

PRACTICE TIPS FOR DOCTORS: DR. JUDITH J. PETRY ON ENGAGING THE BODY'S HEALING RESPONSE

"Whatever we uncover as we explore the illnesses with which we are confronted, our new assumptions about reality allow us to let go of the need to fight the illness, to wage a battle against death, using our bodies as the battlefield. The illness can be engaged in a new way. We can ask our bodies what kind of help we can provide to rebalance in the face of this dis-ease, this disharmony; volunteering all the parts of ourselves, our bodies, our minds, emotions, spirit and community, in this opportunity to reach a higher level of vitality. We can joyfully utilize whatever methods feel life-enhancing and healing to us, including surgery, chemotherapy, radiation, acupuncture, psychotherapy, homeopathy, imagery, nutrition, or any of the other myriad of options available to facilitate our return to wholeness."[7]

Dr. Judith J. Petry, a successful surgeon for sixteen years, is currently medical director of the Vermont Healing Tools Project in Brattleboro, Vermont. The holistic treatment facility employs CAM therapies, like herbs and mind-body relaxation techniques, to ease the pain and anxiety of surgery and speed healing.

the more vulnerable they were to post-op lung infections. Patients who abstained from smoking the longest before surgery had the best outcomes, prompting the authors of the study to recommend that surgery be delayed for at least eight weeks after quitting. Talk to your doctor early about enrolling in a smoking-cessation program.

Ease Up on Alcohol

Heavy drinking suppresses the immune system and may have blood-thinning effects. It stands to reason then that drinking a great deal before surgery could impair healing and raise the risk of infection. In fact, one study showed that moderate-to-heavy drinkers (at least six glasses of wine a day) have twice the risk of post-op infection as other surgical patients.[8] If you're a heavy drinker (more than ten drinks per week), try cutting down in the month before elective surgery. Ideally, consume no alcohol the week before to get your body used to a "dry" state.

Cut Caffeine

Few studies suggest that caffeine itself interferes with surgery or recovery. Granted, some finicky plastic surgeons prefer that patients halt caffeine before surgery, because like nicotine, it's a vasoconstrictor and may interfere with blood flow in tiny vessels and impede healing. And, since caffeine is a mild diuretic, it could theoretically interfere with fluid balance in the all-important recuperation phase. Additionally, excess caffeine can cause arrhythmias and high blood pressure.

But the real reason to limit caffeine before surgery has nothing to do with its potential toxic effects. Rather, it's the *absence* of caffeine—caffeine withdrawal—that makes it advisable. Many patients complain after waking from surgery that they feel like a truck has mowed them down. They're irritable, headachy, and nauseated. Most patients and doctors assume it's just an anesthesia "hangover." But thought-provoking research now suggests that sudden caffeine withdrawal (most coffee drinkers only stop the day before surgery) may be the real culprit.

To prevent flu-like caffeine-withdrawal symptoms (which typically begin twelve to twenty-four hours after your last cup), start gradually tapering off caffeine consumption several weeks before surgery. Begin by eliminating one cup of coffee or soda from your daily ration. With coffee, try a brew of half-caffeinated and half-decaf. If you're a tea drinker, go for shorter brewing times, which cuts down on caffeine content. Or try herbal teas or hot water with lemon. Be sure to drink plenty of water throughout the day. Substitute exercise (a stimulant) for caffeine.

Devise a Nutritional Support Plan

Studies show that your body needs adequate calories and a variety of vitamins and minerals to heal effectively (many are discussed below). For instance, low vitamin C and zinc levels (both necessary to make skin collagen) have been linked to wound separation and poor healing. Increased infection rates are also frequently found in patients with low albumin (protein) levels. This can be compounded during surgery because protein found in red blood cells is typically lost during bleeding. So is iron. The resulting anemia may decrease oxygen delivery to wounds, delay healing, and make you feel weak and tired.

Therefore, I recommend eating a balanced diet in the weeks before surgery (see www.drhoffman.com/page.cfm/21 for more on my Salad and Salmon Diet) and taking some or all of the supplements described below.

TELL YOUR SURGEON ABOUT THESE

The following nutritional supplements can help boost post-surgical healing and cut pain. But be sure to discuss potential side effects with your doctor before taking them.

Acidophilus

Surgery patients often receive antibiotics to prevent infection, especially in gastrointestinal surgery. Whenever antibiotics are taken, though, it's essential to restore the normal balance of intestinal bacteria by also taking probiotics—good bacteria. Imbalances can cause diarrhea, fatigue, suppressed immunity, and yeast infections.

Hospitals are catching up in this regard, often prescribing yogurt with live acidophilus cultures to replenish depleted flora at the time of surgery. I suggest also taking one capsule of *Lactobacillus acidophilus* three times daily before or after antibiotic administration, but not during it.

Arginine

During my years at Albert Einstein College of Medicine, one of my favorite professors was Dr. Sam Seifter who taught biochemistry. I became an even bigger fan after I learned about his "secret" project to prove that a certain nutrient—the amino acid arginine—enhanced surgical outcomes. Research has since confirmed his theory.

In animal studies, oral supplementation with arginine helps delicate skin flaps heal better. When teamed with omega-3s and RNA (a building block for protein synthesis) in an immune-enhancing drink, called IMPACT, arginine also reduces trauma, lowers inflammation, and boosts immune function in patients undergoing surgery for cancer of the gastrointestinal tract.[9] Only 14 percent of patients receiving IMPACT before surgery got post-op infections, compared to over 30 percent of those who didn't drink it. Likewise, the IMPACT group averaged 11.6 days in the hospital versus 14 days for the non-IMPACT group. Other studies show similar benefits for heart-surgery patients who drink IMPACT (see "Revisiting Controversies" on page 208).

Suggested dosage: Prior to surgery, load up on arginine-rich foods, including dairy, meat, poultry and fish, as well as nuts and chocolate. In addition, ask your doctor about IMPACT, or other comparable pre-surgery "cocktails." Or take four to five 1,000-milligram L-arginine capsules, three times daily. Start five days before surgery and continue for three days afterward. (Individuals with recurrent herpes should avoid high doses of L-arginine, which can trigger flares. Likewise, for individuals taking nitroglycerin-type medications or erectile dysfunction drugs).

Bromelain

Derived from the pineapple plant, bromelain is one of many proteolytic enzymes that aid in digestion. Studies show that its anti-inflammatory effects also help reduce post-operative swelling, heal wounds more quickly, and even cut post-surgical pain.

Beginning seventy-two hours before surgery, take 500–1,500 mg of bromelain three or four times a day on an empty stomach. Nature's Plus makes a very good 500-mg bromelain supplement, which delivers 600 gdu (gel dissolving units). You might also try a proteolytic enzyme supplement, such as Wobenzym, which combines bromelain with bioflavonoids like rutin (shown to also reduce swelling), as well as other natural digestive enzymes. Take three to five tablets, two or three times daily, thirty to forty minutes before each meal or not less than sixty minutes after meals.

A few caveats: Don't take bromelain if you're allergic to pineapple. Because it and other proteolytic enzymes have a slight blood-thinning effect, speak to your doctor first if you're taking Coumadin or another anticoagulant.

Fish Oil

As mentioned earlier, omega-3 fatty acids get a bad rap from surgeons because of their blood-thinning properties. However, fish oil taken at lower doses may have distinct benefits in surgery, which likely outweigh its modest, and largely theoretical, bleeding risks.

As we'll see shortly under "Revisiting Controversies," fish oil seems to help heart-surgery patients avoid post-op complications and reduce their hospital stays. Additionally, when combined with L-arginine, it also reduces post-surgical inflammation in patients undergoing colorectal and heart surgery.

Talk to your doctor about taking fish oil before and after surgery. Depending on your risk profile, you may need to either reduce or increase the amount you currently take or discontinue it altogether. For patients who aren't at elevated risk of bleeding, I recommend one capsule of EPA/DHA (1,000 mg) twice daily with food, starting five days before surgery and continuing throughout recovery.

A word of caution: Patients with a hereditary blood disorder, called von Willebrand's syndrome, which occurs in about 1 percent of the population and accentuates the blood-thinning effects of fish oil, should discontinue taking omega-3s prior to surgery. If you bleed excessively when cut or bruise easily, a simple blood test can confirm that you have this syndrome.

Glutamine

When the body is stressed from surgery, steroid hormones, such as cortisol, are released into the bloodstream. Elevated cortisol levels can deplete glutamine stores in the body. Since this amino acid plays a key role in keeping the immune system humming, a deficiency can put the brakes on healing.

Studies have shown that glutamine revs up the immune system, cuts infections, and promotes cell growth and organ repair. It also acts as a building block for production of glutathione, the body's premier antioxidant.

Suggested dosage: 1 teaspoon to 1 tablespoon of L-glutamine powder three times daily, dissolved in cold water. Build up three days prior and continue at least three days after surgery. I typically make use of my own pre-surgical IV "cocktail," which provides high intravenous doses of L-glutamine and other critical nutrients a day or so prior to elective surgery. My patients tend to breeze through surgery and recovery, sometimes astonishing their doctors.

Doctors can learn more about administering these IVs and specific recipes by attending conferences and workshops, including those offered by the American College for Advancement in Medicine (www.acam.org).

Iron

Your surgeon may dismiss your use of arginine and antioxidants, but few surgeons deny that iron is an important pre-op nutrient. Unfortunately, it usually takes three or four months to fully respond to iron supplementation, and most surgeries are booked only a few weeks in advance.

Also, many "natural" iron formulations are too weak to pack a punch. I recommend a newer prescription form of iron called Niferex. Take 150 mg two or three times per day, as far before surgery as possible. Iron is best absorbed with additional vitamin C (500 mg three times daily). Keep in mind, though, that iron can be constipating. For those who can't tolerate it, I recommend a diet high in iron-rich foods. And not just spinach (those Popeye cartoons spawned a lot of misinformation!). Red meat and organ meats are actually preferable to plant sources because they offer more bio-available heme iron.

Tip: Ask your surgeon to check your ferritin levels with a target of 70 ng/ml (nanograms per milliliter) or higher for optimal results (see Chapter 4). Because some patients have excess iron levels, care should be taken to avoid using iron indiscriminately for surgery.

Magnesium

Many of us are low in magnesium, but severe deficiency is most common among debilitated or malnourished patients—the elderly, the poor, and junk-food junkies. Not only can magnesium deficiency predispose surgical patients to heart arrhythmias, but it also makes it harder to "wean" patients off breathing ventilators. No matter your age or nutritional status, supplementing with magnesium is good surgery "insurance."

Suggested dosage: Look for the total *elemental* magnesium in your multivitamin or magnesium supplement (not the weight of the pills, but the actual amount of magnesium they deliver, usually indicated on the label). Take 200–400 mg of elemental magnesium before surgery or as soon after as you can swallow. For heart surgery, or for those with an underlying heart condition, I recommend magnesium taurate.

Vitamin C

This surgical nutrient *par excellence* is essential for synthesis of collagen (which provides structural support and elasticity to the skin). In fact, one hallmark of scurvy (a condition caused by severe vitamin C deficiency) is poor wound healing. C deficiency is also linked to excessive post-op bleeding.

Vitamin C is a crucial antioxidant, as well, and may be part of team of nutrients that can forestall "reperfusion injury" in heart and brain surgery (see "Revisiting Controversies" on page 208).

Suggested dosage: 500 mg of Ester C (an easier form to absorb), three times daily for a week before and a week after surgery. My pre-surgery IV formula also contains generous doses of vitamin C.

Vitamin E

Like fish oil, vitamin E is often shunned by surgeons for its alleged blood-thinning effects. But when combined with other antioxidants like vitamin C, and especially if it's timed to coincide with post-surgical recuperation, vitamin E offers substantial benefits.

The reason may be that surgical complications are brought on, in part, by damage to tissues and organs from free radicals. As we've seen, antioxidants halt this kind of damage. A recent study of 595 critically ill surgical patients admitted to intensive care found that those taking 1,000 IU of vitamin E and 1,000 mg of vitamin C three times a day had far fewer instances of multiple organ failure and were released significantly earlier than those who didn't take these vitamins.[10]

Suggested dosage: 400 IU of mixed tocopherol vitamin E one week prior to surgery and one week after. If you're already taking more before surgery, reduce to 400 IU at least ten days prior to the operation. Resume 800 IU as soon as wound healing begins after post-operative bleeding is under control.

Zinc

Evidence for zinc's importance in wound healing and maintaining optimal immunity comes from research about zinc deficiency. When the body is low in zinc, wounds take longer to close, skin collagen is not as strong, and the immune system has fewer infection-fighting white blood cells. In fact, zinc deficiency is especially common among sick people with poor appetites—precisely those who are earmarked for surgery.

Unfortunately, the stress of surgery and recovery also seems to draw down reserves of zinc. In one study, serum zinc levels dropped by about 46 percent from their pre-op levels.[11]

Therefore, it's particularly important to supplement with zinc before and after surgery. Eat plenty of high-zinc foods, like oysters, nuts, whole grains, meat, and seafood, and take 30 mg of zinc gluconate, picolinate, or sulfate once daily for a week leading up to surgery and during the week afterward.

REVISITING CONTROVERSIES

These controversial therapies are nevertheless promising and worth a second look with your surgeon.

Music Therapy

It's been said that music soothes the savage breast. Apparently, it also eases the rigors of surgery. Years of research suggests that listening to music daily before surgery for a set block of time not only reduces pre-op and post-op jitters, but also decreases post-surgical complications and speeds recovery. Here are just a few of music's healing powers:

- Reduces pre-surgery anxiety, including cutting cortisol levels. Even listening to music for a short time in the surgical holding area before an operation, seems to dramatically diminish stress.

- Listening to music in the days before surgery also lowers heart rate and improves blood pressure and respiration rates *afterward*. Heart patients who receive a combination of music therapy, guided imagery and healing touch are also more likely to stay alive in the months after surgery.

- Music therapy following surgery lowers systolic and diastolic blood pressure, cuts post-op anxiety, boosts mood, reduces reports of pain and lowers the need for pain medications.

- When music is played *during* surgery, patients who receive regional anesthesia and stay awake report that they aren't as aware of the surgical procedure. They also require less anesthesia, stay calmer, and maintain more stable pulse rates and blood pressure.

Though many surgeons remain skeptical about the benefits of music, more and more hospitals are launching music therapy programs. See if your hospital has one or contact the Certification Board for Music Therapists or American Music Therapy Association for names of music therapists in your area (see Resources for Patients).

Arnica: Homeopathy for Surgery?

Arnica montana (a.k.a. "leopard's bane") has been used for hundreds of years to treat inflammation and reduce bruising and swelling. Found growing near Alpine mountain trails, arnica is frequently used by injured hikers and climbers. However, it's more often taken in tincture or pill form, which is homeopathically diluted to contain a very tiny fraction of the dosage available in the raw plant.

When used around the time of surgery, some studies show that arnica reduces bruising and swelling. However, most of these studies weren't closely controlled scientific experiments, and two of the most prominent trials were performed by Alpine Pharmaceuticals, a major manufacturer of arnica with an obvious financial interest in the product.

While many patients and some cosmetic surgeons extol the benefits of arnica, most recent placebo-controlled studies have failed to document its effectiveness. Even so, I believe there's a place for it as an accompaniment to surgery. At the very least, arnica may harness the body's innate healing capacities by engaging the placebo response (a positive reaction to sham medication that the patient believes is real). Take two or three drops of arnica tincture under the tongue three times on the day of surgery and on the day after. Or take five tiny pellets three times on those days.

Acupuncture

Acupuncture became a poster child for the controversy over alternative therapies during the Nixon years in the early 1970s. That was when the first "cultural exchanges" permitted delegations of U.S. doctors to witness surgery in Chinese hospitals. What impressed them most was the pervasive use of traditional Chinese medicine alongside high-tech surgical methods. In well-publicized articles, Americans read about the wonders of acupuncture, which allowed Chinese patients to undergo major surgeries with little or no anesthesia.

However, initial enthusiasm wasn't followed by widespread adoption in American operating rooms. Even so, I believe acupuncture can play an important adjunct role in surgery. For one thing, it appears to combat post-op nausea and vomiting (a problem for almost a quarter of patients who undergo major surgery) better than mainstream anti-nausea drugs.[12] Researchers at Duke University found that just 27 percent of women who received high-tech electroacupuncture during breast surgery complained of sickness afterward, compared to about 50 percent who received the popular anti-nausea drug Zofran and 60 percent who received a sham treatment.

Acupuncture (specifically ear acupuncture or auriculotherapy) also seems to quiet pre-op jitters. The technique involves inserting superfine needles at a specific area of the outer ear, believed to be related to anxiety. One study found that patients who underwent ear acupuncture alone or combined with relaxation techniques were significantly less anxious before elective outpatient surgery than the control group.[13] See Resources for Patients to find qualified acupuncturists.

Nutrient Support for Heart Surgery?

I know the argument: "Sure, taking additional vitamins and bromelain is fine for *minor* surgeries. But when it comes to heavy-duty heart surgery, better lay off!"

All but a handful of heart surgeons (such as forward-thinkers like Mehmet Oz, M.D., profiled below) are wary of using nutritional support for their patients. But what does the research say?

Interestingly, contrary to conventional medical wisdom, supplementing with several antioxidants appears to help rather than hinder the outcome of heart surgery. For instance, fish oil, a potential blood thinner, appears to have a favorable effect when taken at lower dosages. In one recent study, patients receiving omega-3 fatty acids during hospitalization for a coronary artery bypass graft had a 54 percent lower risk of post-op atrial fibrillation (a type of arrhythmia that raises the risk of blood clots) and shorter hospital stays.[14]

Magnesium also reduces atrial fibrillation (see above). In fact, low levels of this mineral are linked to bad outcomes in several heart-surgery studies.

PRACTICE TIP FOR DOCTORS: A PROMINENT HEART SURGEON EXPLORES ALTERNATIVES

Like many holistic physicians, renowned heart surgeon Dr. Mehmet Oz stumbled into the field of complementary and alternative medicine almost by accident. A rising star in the Department of Cardiothoracic Surgery at New York-Presbyterian Hospital/Columbia University Medical Center, Dr. Oz and his colleagues were redesigning a partial artificial heart to keep patients alive while they waited for heart transplants when he had an epiphany. Why not urge anxious patients to try stress-busting alternative approaches at the same time? The results were startling. Not only did patients who tried these therapies, including therapeutic touch, reflexology, music, and hypnotherapy, have less stress and pain during and after surgery, but they also healed more quickly.

This revelation prompted Oz to found Columbia's Integrative Medicine Program in 1994, where he continues to act as medical director. His aim: to combine the high-tech world of ventricular assist devices and mitral-valve repair with holistic healing.

Today, he and his team of CAM healers are at the forefront of studying how complementary approaches boost pre-op and post-op outcomes. Their philosophy centers on treating patients as whole people and not just ailing hearts. Patients choose from any number of promising healing therapies, including free massages from licensed therapists, free weekly post-surgical yoga classes, and music therapy, a particular favorite of Dr. Oz. Learn more in his book *Healing from the Heart: A Leading Heart Surgeon Explores the Power of Complementary Medicine*.

High-risk heart patients who receive the nutrient cocktail IMPACT (combining L-arginine, omega-3s, and RNA) before surgery also appear to benefit.[15] Dutch researchers found that following surgery, only four of twenty-three patients (17 percent) taking the immune-system enhancer developed infection, compared with twelve of the twenty-two patients (55 percent) who received a placebo.

Antioxidants also play a key role in fighting surgery-related free-radical damage. One of the thorniest problems associated with circulation-restoring surgery is ischemia-reperfusion injury. This occurs when blood floods back into an oxygen-starved organ after surgery. Depriving organs of blood flow makes them particularly vulnerable to oxidative damage. Particularly important in fighting this type of free-radical injury are vitamins C and E (discussed earlier), as well as coenzyme Q_{10}. CoQ_{10} has been shown to cut the number of erratic heartbeats patients experience and reduce use of blood pressure drugs. I recommend 150 mg of CoQ_{10} daily before and after surgery.

Ginger for Post-Surgical Nausea

Research is mixed on whether ginger prevents nausea and vomiting following surgery. In some studies, one gram of ginger root before surgery halted nausea as effectively as a leading medication. Other studies, however, have failed to show the same positive effects. In fact, one study found that ginger actually increased vomiting following surgery.

Certainly further studies are needed. However, in my opinion concerns about ginger aren't substantiated in the medical literature. Nor has it posed any problems for my patients. Take 1 tablespoon of compounded ginger syrup, three to four times per day, the day before surgery.

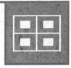

Where We Are,
Where We're Headed

In her book *The Spirit Catches You and You Fall Down*, Anne Fadiman recounts the true story of an immigrant Hmong family in Merced, California in the 1980s whose youngest daughter, Lia, is diagnosed with severe epilepsy.[1] From her doctors' Western medical perspective, Lia's condition is serious but treatable with appropriate medication and high-tech vigilance. For her loving parents, though, Lia's condition represents something else entirely—evidence that her soul, frightened by the slamming of a door, has fled her body and is now lost to a bad spirit (a common explanation for illness in Hmong culture).

What unfolds is a clash of cultures that ultimately ends in tragedy. Both Lia's doctors and parents want the best care possible for her. But the language barrier, plus a lack of cultural understanding and trust, hinders this at every step. As Fadiman notes, "What the doctors viewed as clinical efficiency the Hmong viewed as frosty arrogance."

Lia's parents attempt to supplement her medical treatment with visits to a shaman and animal sacrifices, but are met with disdain from her alarmed doctors. Likewise, her doctors insist on lengthy hospitalizations and a strict regimen of medications, which her parents increasingly resist because they fear treatment is making her worse. The result: Lia is removed from her parents' care by the well-meaning medical community. What follows is a string of devastating missteps and miscommunications with no winners.

Granted, this is an extreme example of what can happen when two medical world-views collide—a classic anthropological standoff between a fierce, insular people who've survived for centuries on the strength of their ancient healing ways and Western doctors who lay their full medical faith at the foot of scientifically scrutinized, technology-based drug and surgical interventions.

The current standoff between mainstream medicine and CAM described throughout these pages isn't on par with the tsunami-like collision recounted by Fadiman. Nor are the consequences of conflict usually so dire. American patients and doctors tend to speak the same language and spring from the same Western healing paradigm. In other words, they at least understand the ground rules and recognize where the other is coming from. Few patients insist on retrieving their kidnapped souls from evil spirits by offering up the souls of slaughtered pigs as barter. Nor do most doctors forcibly remove patients from their homes and families to ensure they follow prescribed care plans.

Even so, perspective is often gained by stepping back and observing one's situation impartially—through the anthropologist's lens, if you will. From that vantage point, the scuffle between CAM and mainstream medicine shares many similarities with Fadiman's tale. Lack of trust, lack of compliance with care recommendations, lack of satisfaction, and suboptimal care are all part of the shift taking place in American medicine. Disagreements between doctors and patients may center on little more than whether to enhance chemotherapy with nutritional supplements. But the fallout often leaves both sides scratching their heads, or worse, exhausted and bitter. "Why won't my doctor listen and work with me on this?" patients wonder. "Why can't patients respect my expert medical opinion and leave the decisions to me?" doctors complain.

Yet I'm hopeful that this shift, however difficult, is moving us all toward a true integration of mainstream medicine and CAM. Just as Lia's parents fought for her right to use a blend of Western drugs and Hmong folk rituals and herbs—for her to be seen as a whole person and not just a set of symptoms—many patients today are seeking these same health freedoms. At least one new study, published in *Diabetes Care,* supports this notion.[2] Researchers found that contrary to most doctors' fears, diabetics who use CAM therapies, such as acupuncture, chiropractic care, herbal therapy, or relaxation therapy (a surprising 48 percent now rely on these adjunct approaches) are actually more likely to also use conventional medical treatments than to shun them. The authors noted that patients appear to want autonomy to use the best of both medical worlds rather than rely on a single approach.

It seems we all want—and should have the right—to follow our unique healing paths, which may mean intertwining proven high-tech treatments with proven CAM modalities. We want our doctor's blessing, but also his or her expert guidance. We want a holistic approach to our care.

Doctors are also seeking better relationships with patients and are waking up to the promise of CAM. They recognize increasingly that good care means using the full range of effective treatments at their disposal. And they know that the best medicine requires allying themselves with patients and listening to their needs.

In the following sections, you'll find a chapter-by-chapter listing of important patient resources, plus citations for evidence-based CAM studies discussed throughout this book. These should help you craft the care you want and hopefully communicate more effectively and intelligently with your doctor. Sharing them could lead to a more honest and open dialog, plus it might also bolster your case for incorporating CAM therapies.

Doctors will also find an extensive list of physician resources, including reputable professional organizations and educational opportunities, to help them better understand the kind of integrative care patients are seeking and encourage them to take a more holistic approach to health care. My hope is that these resources and the information laid out in this book will help to further expand our medical choices and foster stronger doctor-patient partnerships.

Resources
for Patients

While every effort has been made to include the most up-to-date information at the time of publication, be aware that the following addresses, telephone numbers, e-mail addresses, and website links are subject to change.

Chapter 1: Why Doctors Act the Way They Do

Books

Konner, Melvin. *Becoming a Doctor: A Journey of Initiation in Medical School,* New York, NY: Penguin, 1987.

Marion, Robert. *Learning to Play God,* New York, NY: Fawcett, 2000.

Chapter 2: Medicine and Health Care in Flux

Articles/Reports

"To Err Is Human: Building a Safer Health System." Report by Committee on Quality of Health Care in America, Institute of Medicine of the National Academies (2000): www.nap.edu/catalog/9728.html.

Books

Murcott, Toby. *The Whole Story: Alternative Medicine on Trial?* London, England: Palgrave Macmillan, 2005.

Chapter 3: Creating a New Vision of Medical Practice

Articles/Reports

Sierpina, Victor S. "Teaching Integratively: How the Next Generation of Doctors Will Practice." *Integrative Cancer Therapies* Vol. 3, No. 3 (2004): pp. 201–207.

Books

Dossey, Larry. *Reinventing Medicine: Beyond Mind-Body to a New Era of Healing,* San Francisco, CA: Harper, 1999.

Franklin, Tel. *Expect a Miracle, You Won't Be Disappointed,* Monterey, CA: Center for Appreciative Medicine, 2003. Book orders: http://www.appreciativemedicine.com or call (800) 641-7771.

Hoffman, Ronald. *Natural Therapies for Mitral Valve Prolapse,* New Canaan, CT: Keats Publishing, Inc., 1997. Book orders: www.drhoffman.com/page.cfm/327 or call (800) 456-9384.

Neuman, Fredric. *Worried Sick? The Exaggerated Fear of Physical Illness,* Larchmont, NY: Hadrian Press, 2003.

Your Daily Diary & Health Journal: Helping You Live Your Best Life, Laguna Beach, CA: Basic Health Publications, 2004.

Newsletters on Alternative Therapies

Alternative Medicine Alert: www.altmednet.com/titles/ama.html. Monthly newsletter providing clinicians and patients with evidence-based information on alternative and complementary therapies. Published by Thomson American Health Consultants.

Dr. Andrew Weil's Self Healing Newsletter: www.drweilselfhealing.com. Information on integrative medicine and health tips from holistic physician Andrew Weil, M.D.

Health & Healing: www.drwhitaker.com/c/store_hh_prod2.asp. Monthly newsletter on natural therapies by holistic physician Julian Whitaker, M.D.

Holistic Primary Care: News for Health and Healing: www.holisticprimarycare.net. Online and print publication for physicians and general public, offering scientific information on holistic medicine.

Townsend Letter for Doctors & Patients: www.townsendletter.com. Balanced, scientific information on variety of alternative medicine topics.

Organizations

American Botanical Council: www.herbalgram.org or (800) 373-7105. Provides news, searchable databases, and latest scientific research on herbal medicines.

Consortium of Academic Health Centers for Integrative Medicine: www.imconsortium.org. Organization of academic medical centers offering integrative education, research, and care.

National Center for Complementary and Alternative Medicine: www.nccam.nih.gov/health or (888) 644-6226. A division of the National Institutes of Health. Provides articles and databases of latest CAM research.

Web-based Health Information

Consumer Lab: www.consumerlab.com. Provides independent test results on hundreds of vitamins, herbs and natural products to help consumers and doctors evaluate their nutritional content.

Council for Responsible Nutrition: www.crnusa.org. 1828 L Street, NW, Suite 900, Washington, D.C., 20036-5114; (202) 776-7929. Scientific information on vitamin and herbal supplements.

HealthFinder: www.healthfinder.gov. Consumer friendly articles, organizations and links from the Department of Health and Human Services.

Health on the Net Foundation: www.hon.ch. An international non-profit organization of medical experts that accredits health websites through its "Code of Conduct" standards. Lists accredited sites.

Holistic Healing Web Page: www.holisticmed.com. A treasure trove of alternative/holistic medicine topics and resources with articles, conference listings, discussion groups, and disease databases.

International Bibliographic Information on Dietary Supplements (IBIDS) Database: http://ods.od. nih.gov/Health_Information/IBIDS.aspx. A service of the National Institutes of Health Office of Dietary Supplements, offering citations and abstracts from scientific literature on dietary supplements.

Internet Resources—Alternative Medicine Resources: www.pitt.edu/~cbw/internet.html. Offers hundreds of resources and links on specific diseases, nutrition, mind-body therapies, government resources, vitamins and much more.

MayoClinic.com: www.mayohealth.org. Good resource for general information about specific conditions, like Alzheimer's disease and cancer.

MedicineNet: www.medicinenet.com. News, health updates, and searchable medical dictionary.

Medline Plus: www.nlm.nih.gov/medlineplus. A service of the National Library of Medicine and the National Institutes of Health, providing information on over 650 diseases and conditions, lists of hospitals and physicians, a medical encyclopedia and medical dictionary, information on prescription and nonprescription drugs, links to thousands of clinical trials and ability to search for studies on MedLine.

National Guideline Clearinghouse: www.guideline.gov. Primarily for health professionals, but patients can research recommended treatments for hundreds of conditions.

PatientInform: www.patientinform.org/PI/home.jsp. Free online service from leading medical associations providing access to and analysis of up-to-date, reliable research on the diagnosis and treatment of specific diseases.

PubMed: www.ncbi.nlm.nih.gov/entrez/query.fcgi. A service of the National Library of Medicine, which includes public access to MedLine, provides citations for over 15 million studies.

PubMed CAM-related articles: www.nlm.nih.gov/nccam/camonpubmed.html.

UpToDate: www.uptodate.com. Latest peer-reviewed mainstream treatment guidelines for hundreds of conditions, updated on continuous basis. Section for physicians and patients allows collaboration on treatment plan.

VitaSearch: www.vitasearch.com. Free literature search on any health topic.

Chapter 4: Getting a Real Physical Exam
Body Mass Index

National Heart, Lung and Blood Institute online Body Mass Index calculator: http://nhlbisupport. com/bmi/bmicalc.htm.

Books

Braly, James and Ron Hoggan. *Dangerous Grains: Why Gluten Cereal Grains May Be Hazardous to Your Health,* New York, NY: Avery Publishing Group, 2002.

Brodin, Michael. *The Encyclopedia of Medical Tests,* New York, NY: Pocket Books, 1997.

Hoffman, Ronald. *Intelligent Medicine,* New York, NY: Fireside, 1997. Book orders: www. drhoffman.com/page.cfm/293 or call (800) 456-9384.

Hoffman, Ronald. *Natural Therapies for Mitral Valve Prolapse,* New Canaan, CT: Keats Publishing, Inc., 1997. Book orders: www.drhoffman.com/page.cfm/327 or call (800) 456-9384.

Perricone, Nicholas. *The Wrinkle Cure: Unlock the Power of Cosmeceuticals for Supple, Youthful Skin,* New York, NY: Warner Books, 2000.

Theodosakis, Jason and David T. Feinberg. *Don't Let Your HMO Kill You: How to Wake Up Your Doctor, Take Control of Your Health, and Make Managed Care Work For You,* New York, NY: Routledge, 2000.

Zaret, Barry, Peter Jatlow and Lee Katz. *The Yale University School of Medicine Patient's Guide to Medical Tests,* Boston, MA: Houghton Mifflin, 1997.

Celiac Sprue Disease

Celiac Sprue Association: www.csaceliacs.org (for patients). P.O. Box 31700 Omaha, NE 68131-0700; (877) CSA-4CSA (4272).

Environmental Medicine

American Academy of Environmental Medicine: www.aaem.com. 7701 East Kellogg, Suite 625, Wichita, KS 67207; (316) 684-5500.

"Body Burden Report," *Mount Sinai School of Medicine, Environmental Working Group & Commonweal* (January 2003): www.ewg.org/reports/bodyburden/es.php.

Center for Children's Health and the Environment: www.childenvironment.org. Mount Sinai School of Medicine, P.O. Box 1043, 1 Gustave Levy Place, New York, NY 10029; (212) 241-7840. Examines link between childhood disease and exposure to pollutants.

Collaborative on Health and the Environment: www.healthandenvironment.org. c/o Commonweal, P.O. Box 316, Bolinas, CA 94924. Involved in education and prevention of disease via environmental factors.

"National Report on Human Exposure to Environmental Chemical" (Reports 1, 2, & 3). *Centers for Disease Control and Prevention.* March 2001, January 2003 & July 2005: www.cdc.gov/exposurereport/.

Science and Environmental Health Network: www.sehn.org. PMB 282 217 Welch Ave. Suite 101 Ames, IA 50014; (515) 268-0600. Focuses on environmental health issues, such as biotechnology and reproductive and developmental toxins.

Medical Testing Labs

Consumer Lab: www.consumerlab.com. Provides independent test results on hundreds of vitamins, herbs, and natural products to help consumers and doctors evaluate their nutritional content.

Doctor's Data, Inc.: www.doctorsdata.com. An independent reference laboratory providing data on levels of toxic and essential elements in hair, and elements, amino acids, and metabolites in blood and urine. For information on tests and services, call (800) 323-2784.

Genova Diagnostics: www.gdx.net. Offers full range of clinical tests, including for hormonal, allergic, and other conditions; (800) 522-4762.

BodyBalance: www.bodybalance.com. Consumer division, offers testing kits directly to consumers, including hormonal and bone density tests; (888) 891-3061.

Immunosciences Lab, Inc.: www.immuno-sci-lab.com/index2.html.Develops esoteric tests and helps clinicians in the diagnosis of very complex diseases where the immune system is directly or indirectly involved; (800) 950-4686.

Lab Tests Online: http://labtestsonline.org/site/index.html. Provides hundreds of lab test descriptions and recommended tests for specific conditions.

Metametrix Clinical Laboratory: www.metametrix.com. Offers a full range of tests, including metabolic profiles, hormone profiles, and oxidative stress indicators. For information on tests and services, call (800) 221-4640.

Paying for Medical Tests

Dr. Jason Theodosakis's website: www.drtheo.com. Includes forms to assist in writing letters of appeal when insurance companies won't pay for medical tests.

Recommendations for Routine Preventive Tests

Park Nicollet Health Advisor's Check-up Schedule: www.parknicollet.com/healthadvisor/checkupschedule/recommendations_2.cfm.

- **Ages Nineteen to Thirty-Nine**

When to Schedule a Visit

It is recommended that men see their doctor every five years for a complete preventive care visit. Women should schedule a visit every three to five years. Each visit includes a height and weight check, blood pressure check, preventive counseling, health risk assessment, and any necessary screening tests or immunizations. Blood pressure checks may need to be done more often.

Screening Tests

Men and Women

- Blood pressure check: Every two years

Men

- Cholesterol check: Every five years beginning at age thirty-five

Women

- Clinical breast examination: Every three years beginning at age twenty
- Pap test and pelvic examination: Every three years (after three consecutive, annual, normal tests)

- **Ages Forty to Sixty-Four**

When to Schedule a Visit

It is recommended that men see their doctor every five years for a complete preventive care visit. Women should schedule a visit every three to five years. Each visit includes a height and weight check, blood pressure check, preventive counseling, health risk assessment, and any other necessary screening tests or immunizations. Blood pressure checks, influenza vaccinations, clinical breast examinations, and mammograms may need to be done more often.

Screening Tests

Men and Women

- Blood pressure check: Every two years
- Cholesterol check: Men, every five years; women, every five years beginning at age forty-five
- Colon cancer screening beginning at age fifty
- Influenza vaccine: every year beginning at age fifty

Women

- Clinical breast examination: Every year
- Mammogram: Every year ages forty to forty-nine: every two years after age fifty (depending on your health history or preference; discuss with your provider)
- Pap test and pelvic examination: Every three years (after three consecutive, annual, normal tests)

- **Ages Sixty-Five and Older**

When to Schedule a Visit

It is recommended that men and women see their doctor every one to two years for a complete preventive care visit. Each visit includes a height and weight check, blood pressure check, preventive counseling, health-risk assessment, and any necessary screening tests or immunizations.

Screening Tests

Men and Women

- Blood pressure check: Every one to two years
- Cholesterol check: Every five years until age seventy-five
- Flexible sigmoidoscopy: Every five years until age eighty
- Hearing and vision screening: Beginning at age seventy-five

Women

- Clinical breast examination: Every year
- Mammogram: Every year until age seventy-five
- Pap test and pelvic examination: Every three years (if regular screening has been done and Pap tests have been normal, screening may be deferred after age sixty-five if patient wishes)

Vitamin D

Vitamin D Council. Facts, articles, and studies on importance of vitamin D: www.cholecalciferol-council.com.

Chapter 5: What to Do When You're Chronically Ill

Books

Ettinger, Alan B. and Deborah M. Weisbrot. *The Essential Patient Handbook: Getting the Health Care You Need—From Doctors Who Know,* New York, NY: Demos Medical Publishing, 2004.

Fink, John M. *Third Opinion: An International Resource Guide to Alternative Therapy Centers for Treating and Preventing Cancer, Arthritis, Diabetes, HIV/AIDS, MS, CFS, and Other Diseases, 4th edition,* Garden City Park, NY: Square One Publishers, 2004.

Fitzpatrick, Margaret, Linda Burke, Daryl Lee. *What to Ask the Doc: The Questions to Ask to Get the Answers You Need,* RN Interactive, Inc., 2003.

Vagnini, Frederic and Barry Fox. *The Side Effects Bible: The Dietary Solution to Unwanted Side Effects of Common Medications,* New York, NY: Broadway, 2005.

Chronic Disease

National Center for Chronic Disease Prevention and Health Promotion

Chronic Disease Prevention: www.cdc.gov/nccdphp. Provides chronic disease statistics and information about specific CDC programs for preventing and treating individual diseases.

Clinical Trials

ClinicalTrials.gov.: http://clinicaltrials.gov. A service of the National Institutes of Health lists thousands of current clinical trials and contact information for participation.

CenterWatch Clinical Trials Listing Service: www.centerwatch.com. Similar service with names of experimental drugs under investigation and recent FDA approvals.

Drug-Nutrient Interactions

Drug-Nutrient Workshop: www.nutritionworkshop.com. Applied Nutrition, Inc., 133 East 73 St., Suite 308, New York, NY 10021. User-friendly tool now available for consumers to view documented or hypothetical reactions that might occur when conventional drugs are combined with herbs, vitamins and minerals, or other supplements.

Center for Food-Drug Interaction Research and Education: www.druginteractioncenter.org. New online tool with patient section to check interactions. Offered by the University of Florida and Tufts University.

Drug and Food Information: www.cc.nih.gov/ccc/patient_education/drug_nutrient. National Institutes of Health Clinical Center, Drug-Nutrient Interaction Task Force. Provides information on specific known drug-food interactions.

Medical Dictionaries

All Health Net list of online medical dictionaries: www.allhealthnet.com/meddict.htm.

MedicineNet's MedTerms Medical Dictionary: www.medterms.com/script/main/hp.asp.

Medline Plus Medical Dictionary: www.nlm.nih.gov/medlineplus/mplusdictionary.html.

Medical Jargon

Partnership for Clear Health Communciation: www.askme3.org. Helps patients and doctors cut through "medicalese."

Narrative Medicine

Charon, Rita. "Narrative Medicine." University of Alaska Anchorage, *LitSite Alaska* website: http://litsite.alaska.edu/healing/medicine.html.

Referrals to Holistic Practitioners

American Academy of Medical Acupuncture: www.medicalacupuncture.org. 4929 Wilshire Boulevard, Suite 428, Los Angeles, California 90010; (323) 937-5514. Free online search for physician acupuncturists in your area.

American Association of Naturopathic Physicians: www.naturopathic.org. 4435 Wisconsin Ave., NW, Suite 403, Washington, D.C. 20016; (866) 538-2267. Free online search for naturopathic physicians offering holistic approach to health care.

American Board of Holistic Medicine: www.holisticboard.org. 1135 Makawao Ave., #230, Makawao, HI 96768; (808) 572-4616. Free referrals to over 650 M.D.s and D.O.s who are board-certified holistic physicians.

American College for Advancement in Medicine: www.acam.org. 23121 Verdugo Dr., Ste 204, Laguna Hills, CA 92653: (888) 439-6891.Free online and phone referrals to more than 1,000 licensed holistic M.D. and D.O. members.

American Holistic Health Association's Resource and Referral List http://ahha.org/ahre.htm. Lists professional organizations that provide referrals to qualified CAM practitioners.

American Holistic Medical Association: www.holisticmedicine.org. 12101 Menaul Blvd., NE, Suite C, Albuquerque, NM 87112; (505) 292-7788. Free online search or send $15 for directory of over 700 holistic M.D.s, D.O.s, and other holistic health providers with current unrestricted licenses.

Institute for Functional Medicine: www.functionalmedicine.org. 411 Pt. Fosdick Drive NW, Suite 305, P.O. Box 1697, Gig Harbor, WA 98335; (800) 228-0622. Free online search for functional medicine doctor in your area.

Second Opinions

American College of Surgeons: "Should You Seek a Consultation (Second Opinion)": www.facs.org/public_info/operation/consult.html.

Cancerdecisions.com: Critically evaluates and contrasts *both* conventional and alternative cancer therapies. For an additional fee, patients can purchase *The Moss Reports,* an individualized summary of various options applicable to their cancer, culled from a database of numerous cancer conditions: www.cancerdecisions.com.

Cancer Second Opinions: www.cancersupportivecare.com/second_opinions.html. Offers several articles by M.D.s on whether second opinions are always necessary and the value they offer.

Mayo Clinic Treatment Decisions: www.mayoclinic.com/health/TreatmentDecisionIndex/TreatmentDecisionIndex.Online tool that helps you and your doctor sort the pros and cons of treatments for problems, such as uterine fibroids and breast cancer, and decide the best healing path for you.

National Women's Health Information Center: How to Get a Second Opinion: www.4woman.gov/tools/SecondOpinion.htm.

Second Opinion Medical Information Services: www.physicians-background.com. For a fee, conducts background checks on doctors, provides list of other possible diagnoses, and locates best hospitals for treatment; (850) 862-5075.

Symptom Guides

AllRefer.com Symptoms Guide: http://health.allrefer.com/health/symptoms.html. Includes step-by-step instructions for evaluating various symptoms.

MyElectronicMD.com: www.myelectronicmd.com. Online self-screening tool allows users to click on area of the body experiencing symptoms to learn about possible underlying causes and best course of action.

WebMD Symptom Checker: http://my.webmd.com/medical_information/check_symptoms/default.htm?z=1727_00000_1110_dp_03. Similar online self-screening tool allowing users to click on body parts with symptoms and sift through possible causes.

Chapter 6: Heart Disease

Chelation Therapy

Chelation Therapy Study: http://nccam.nih.gov/chelation. Sponsored by the National Center for Complementary and Alternative Medicine and the National Heart Lung and Blood Institute; call (888) 644-6226 to see if you're eligible to participate in the study.

American College for Advancement in Medicine: www.acam.org. 23121 Verdugo Dr., Ste 204, Laguna Hills, CA 92653; (888) 439-6891. Free online and phone referrals to more than 1,000 licensed holistic M.D. and D.O. members who practice chelation therapy.

Coenzyme Q_{10}

International Coenzyme Q_{10} Association: www.coenzymeQ10.it/home.html. Provides articles, research summaries, and study citations on CoQ_{10}.

Fish Oil/ Omega-3 Essential Fatty Acids

Omega-3 fatty acid content of various fish and supplements: http://circ.ahajournals.org/cgi/content/full/106/21/2747/TBL3. From the American Heart Association scientific statement on fish consumption, fish oil, omega-3 fatty acids, and heart disease.

Consumer Lab: www.consumerlab.com. Rates fish-oil supplements, concluding that most are free of mercury and chemical contaminants.

Essential Fatty Acid information: www.drhoffman.com/Downloads/Stdv3-2FattyAcids.pdf.

Got Mercury: www.gotmercury.org. Sponsored by the Turtle Island Restoration Project. Allows you to measure whether your mercury intake from fish exceeds EPA limits.

Seafood Choices Alliance: www.seafoodchoices.org. Information on making environmentally friendly, safe seafood choices, including SeaSense database, describing pros and cons of eating several types of sea fish.

Heart Healthy Nutrition and Diet Information

Council for Responsible Nutrition: www.crnusa.org. 1828 L Street, NW, Suite 900, Washington, D.C., 20036-5114; (202) 776-7929. Scientific information on vitamin and herbal supplements.

The Salad and Salmon Diet: www.drhoffman.com/page.cfm/21.

Homocysteine

McCully, Kilmer. *The Heart Revolution: The B Vitamin Breakthrough That Lowers Homocysteine, Cuts Your Risk of Heart Disease, and Protects Your Health,* New York, NY: HarperCollins, 1999.

Homocysteine.net. A wealth of information: www.homocysteine.net/pages/homocysteine/1/abouthcy.html.

Hormone Replacement Therapy

American College for Advancement in Medicine: www.acam.org. 23121 Verdugo Dr., Suite 204, Laguna Hills, CA 92653: (888) 439-6891. For practitioners trained in natural hormone replacement.

College Pharmacy: www.collegepharmacy.com. Compounding pharmacy specializing in natural, customized HRT therapies; (800) 888-9358.

Kronos Early Estrogen Prevention Study (KEEPS), Kronos Longevity Research Institute: www.kronosinstitute.org or www.keepstudy.org; (866) 878-1221.

Postmenopausal Estrogen/Progestin Intervention (PEPI) Trials: www.clinicaltrials.gov/ct/show/NCT00000466.

Testosterone Effects on Atherosclerosis in Aging Men (TEAAM Study): www.kronosinstitute.org/testosterone.htm. Kronos Longevity Research Institute; (866) 878-1221.

Women's Health Initiative: www.nhlbi.nih.gov/whi/index.html. National Heart Lung and Blood Institute.

Women's International Pharmacy: www.womensinternational.com. Compounding pharmacy, specializing in natural, customized HRT therapies; (800) 279-5708.

Hypertension

National Institutes of Health hypertension information page: www.nhlbi.nih.gov/health/dci/Diseases/Hbp/HBP_WhatIs.html.

Magnesium

Dean, Carolyn. *The Miracle of Magnesium* New York, NY: Ballantine Publishing Group, 2003.

Meditation

Meditation Internet Resources: www.holisticmed.com/www/meditation.html. Offers links to dozens of meditation organizations, practitioner databases, education programs and publications.

Transcendental Meditation Program: www.tm.org. Website offers meditation techniques and over 500 studies about the health and brain benefits of meditating.

Nutrigenomics

NutraGenomics, Inc.: www.nutragenomics.com. Research and development bio-technology company devoted to studying nutritional solutions to chronic diseases.

Challem, Jack. *Feed Your Genes Right,* Hoboken, NJ: John Wiley & Sons, 2005.

Strength Training

Centers for Disease Control and Prevention. "Growing Stronger—Strength Training for Older Adults": www.cdc.gov/nccdphp/dnpa/physical/growing_stronger/.

Fitness Over Fifty: An Exercise Guide from the National Institute on Aging, New York, NY: W.W. Norton & Co., 2003.

Westcott, Wayne L. and Thomas R. Baechle, *Strength Training Past 50* (Ageless Athlete Series), Champaign, IL: Human Kinetics Publishers, 1998.

Westcott, Wayne L. "Strength Training for Older Adults." Article on HealthWorld Online: www.healthy.net/scr/article.asp?ID=330.

Westcott, Wayne L. "Twelve Reasons Every Adult Should Do Strength Exercise." Article on HealthWorld Online: www.healthy.net/scr/article.asp?ID=296.

Vitamin E

Council for Responsible Nutrition: www.crnusa.org/vitaminEissafe.html. Discussions on vitamin E safety and flaws in *Annals of Internal Medicine* meta-analysis.

Chapter 7: Cancer

Books

Labriola, Dan. *Complementary Cancer Therapies: Combining Traditional and Alternative Approaches for the Best Possible Outcome,* Roseville, CA: Prima Lifestyles, 2000.

Moss, Ralph W. *Questioning Chemotherapy: A Critique of the Use of Toxic Drugs in the Treatment of Cancer,* Brooklyn, NY: Equinox Press, 1995.

Sontag, Susan. *Illness as Metaphor,* New York, NY: Farrar, Straus & Giroux, 1978.

Cancer Pain

"Facts About Cancer Pain, Part 2: Non-Drug Treatments for Pain." Supplement to *Alternative Medicine Alert* Vol. 8 No. 3 (March 2005): Pages S1–S4. To subscribe visit: www.altmednet.com/titles/ama.html.

Cancer Support Groups

People Living with Cancer: www.plwc.org. Website of the American Society of Clinical Oncology with information on fifty types of cancer, clinical trials, treatment side effects, live chats with experts, and patient support groups.

Cancer Treatment

Cancerdecisions.com: www.cancerdecisions.com. Dr. Ralph W. Moss's website that critically evaluates and contrasts *both* conventional and alternative cancer therapies. Offers cancer treatment tips, free newsletter and area for health professionals. For an additional fee, patients can purchase *The Moss Reports,* an individualized summary of various options applicable to their cancer, culled from a database of numerous cancer conditions.

Cancer Treatment Centers of America: www.cancercenter.com. Network of cancer treatment hospitals that encourage use of CAM approaches, along with conventional cancer therapies; (800) 615-3055.

Curcumin

Curcumin 95: www.jarrow.com. Supplements available from Jarrow Formulas, Inc.; (800) 726-0886.

EGCG Ultra

Order at www.drhoffman.com/page.cfm/278 or (800) 456-9384.

Green Tea with EGCG

Stash brand: www.stashtea.com.

Lycopene

Lycomato supplements: www.lycomato.com; (866) LYCOMATO (592-6628).

PhytoGuard

Order at www.drhoffman.com/page.cfm/341 or (800) 456-9384.

Second Opinions

Cancer Second Opinions: www.cancersupprotivecare.com/second_opinions.html.

Vitamin D

Vitamin D Council: http://www.cholecalciferol-council.com.

Zyflamend

To find a store near you, go to: www.new-chapter.com.

Chapter 8: Arthritic Diseases

Acupuncture

National Certification Commission for Acupuncture and Oriental Medicine: www.nccaom.org/home.htm. Online directory of practitioners certified in acupuncture, Oriental medicine, Chinese herbology and Asian bodywork therapy. 11 Canal Center Plaza, Suite 300, Alexandria, VA 22314; (703) 548-9004.

Boswellin

Boswelya Plus: www.ayush.com. Available from Ayush Herbs, Inc.; (800) 925-1371.

Cat's Claw

Cat's Claw Max D: www.douglaslabs.com. Available from Douglas Laboratories via doctor's offices only; (888) 368-4522.

DHEA/Testosterone

American College for Advancement in Medicine: www.acam.org. 23121 Verdugo Dr., Suite 204, Laguna Hills, CA 92653; (888) 439-6891. For practitioners trained in natural hormone replacement.

College Pharmacy: www.collegepharmacy.com. Compounding pharmacy specializing in natural, customized HRT therapies; (800) 888-9358.

Life Extension Foundation: www.lef.org/protocols/prtcl-130.shtml. Information on natural hormone replacement for men.

Women's International Pharmacy: www.womensinternational.com. Compounding pharmacy, specializing in natural, customized HRT therapies; (800) 279-5708.

Exercise/Swimming

Hydrotherapy Exercises for Arthritis Sufferers: http://arthritis.about.com/od/hydrotherapy/.

Questions and Answers about Arthritis and Exercise: www.niams.nih.gov/hi/topics/arthritis/arthexfs.htm. National Institute of Arthritis and Musculoskeletal and Skin Diseases.

Yoga Therapy for Arthritis: www.yogabasics.com/yogatherapy/arthritis.html. Website with numerous articles, resources, and links.

Extracorporeal Shock Wave Therapy (ESWT)

Excellence Shock Wave Therapy: www.eswtusa.com. Training and credentialing organization that provides ESWT training to physicians. Also, includes information on this non-invasive, drugless pain relief treatment for consumers.

Extracorporeal Shock Wave Therapy Resources: http://heelspurs.com/eswt/index.html. Information about ESWT and journal articles supporting its use.

Glucosamine/Chondroitin

Avosoy. Supplements developed by Jason Theodosakis, M.D., containing glucosamine, chondroitin and ASU (avocado and soy unsaponifiables): order at www.avosoy.com.

Jason Theodosakis, M.D. website: www.drtheo.com. Useful resource for doctors and patients, listing over a dozen peer-reviewed studies that document the effectiveness of glucosamine and/or chondroitin for arthritis.

Theodosakis, Jason, Brenda Adderly, and Barry Fox. *The Arthritis Cure: The Medical Miracle That Can Halt, Reverse, and May Even Cure Osteoarthritis,* New York, NY: Affinity Communications, 1998.

Glycemic Index

The Glycemic Index: www.glycemicindex.com. Offers a database of foods with their glycemic measures from the University of Sydney in Australia.

Lactoferrin

Body Gard with Lactoferrin: Order supplements from The Right Solution at www.rightsolution. com/product_pages/body_gard.html or (702) 317-2400.

Laktoferrin with Colostrum: Order supplements from the Allergy Research Group at www.allergy researchgroup.com/proddesc/category/immune.htm or (800) 545-9960.

Low-Purine Foods

Low-Purine Diet: www.healthsquare.com/mc/fgmc2005.htm. Offers list of low- and high-purine foods.

Magnet Therapy

Nikken Corporation: www.nikken.com. Offers several magnet products for pain relief.

Natural COX-2 Inhibitors

Curcumin 95: Order supplements from Jarrow Formulas, Inc. at www.jarrow.com or (800) 726-0886.

EGCG Ultra: Order at www.drhoffman.com/page.cfm/278 or (800) 456-9384.

Zyflamend: Order from New Chapter Inc.at www.new-chapter.com.

Wobenzym. Order supplements from Naturally Vitamins at www.naturally.com or www.wobenzym.com; or call (888) 766-4406.

Salad and Salmon Diet

Visit: www.drhoffman.com/page.cfm/21.

Stress Relief/Relaxation

American Institute of Stress: www.stress.org/about.htm. Clearinghouse for stress information.

Stress Management and Emotional Wellness Links: http://imt.net/%7Erandolfi/StressLinks.html. Dozens of links to stress management resources from Optimal Health Concepts.

Stress Relief Strategies: www.holisticmed.com/stressfree.html. Good overview of severe stress reduction techniques and resources to learn more.

Undenatured Collagen Type II

Rheumashield: Available from Douglas Laboratories via doctor's offices only at www.douglas labs.com or (888) 368-4522.

Vitamin D and Sun Exposure

Holick, Michael and Mark Jenkins. *The UV Advantage,* iBooks, 2004.

Chapter 9: Cognitive Problems

Articles

QualityCounts.com—Comprehensive Anti-Aging Research: http://qualitycounts.com/fpmemory. html. Treasure-trove of articles on cognitive decline and memory loss.

Life Extension: "Age-Associated Mental Impairment." Excellent introductory discussion at www.lef.org/protocols/prtcl-003.shtml.

Books

Goldberg, Elkhonon, *The Wisdom Paradox: How Your Mind Can Grow Stronger as Your Brain Grows Older,* New York, NY: Gotham Books, 2005.

Coenzyme Q$_{10}$

Vitaline Coenzyme Q$_{10}$: Available only to medical professionals from Vitaline at www. vitaline.com or (800) 931-1709.

Curcumin

Curcumin 95. Available from Jarrow Formulas at www.jarrow.com or (800) 726-0886.

Hormone Replacement Therapy

American College for Advancement in Medicine: www.acam.org. 23121 Verdugo Dr., Suite 204, Laguna Hills, CA 92653; (888) 439-6891. For practitioners trained in natural hormone replacement.

College Pharmacy: www.collegepharmacy.com. Compounding pharmacy specializing in natural, customized HRT therapies; (800) 888-9358.

Women's Health Initiative: www.nhlbi.nih.gov/whi/index.html. National Heart Lung and Blood Institute.

Women's International Pharmacy: www.womensinternational.com. Compounding pharmacy, specializing in natural, customized HRT therapies; (800) 279-5708.

Meditation

Transcendental Meditation Program: www.tm.org. Website offers meditation techniques and over 500 studies about the health and brain benefits of meditating.

Neurotransmitters

NeuroScience Inc.: www.neurorelief.com. Specializes in the assessment and correction of neurotransmitters and hormones. Provides testing, therapeutic and technical support; (888) 342-7272.

Niferex

Manufactured by Ther-Rx Corporation. For more information, contact: www.ther-rx.com or (877) 567-7676.

Drugs.com Prescription Drug Information for Consumers & Professionals: www.drugs.com/niferex. html. Provides information on side effects, dosage, and potential interactions with other drugs.

PS (Phosphatidylserine) and PC (Phosphatidylcholine)

NT Factor. Available at www.ntfactor.com or www.drhoffman.com/page.cfm/332; or call (800) 456-9384.

Chapter 10: Dealing with Diseases That Aren't Diseases

Chronic Fatigue Syndrome

Hoffman, Ronald. *Tired All the Time: How to Regain Your Lost Energy,* New York, NY: Simon and Schuster, 1993.

Cognitive Behavior Therapy (CBT)

Cognitive Behavior Therapy website: www.cognitivetherapy.com. Provides resources, articles and a database of CBT professionals.

Depression

National Institute of Mental Health: www.nimh.nih.gov/publicat/depression.cfm. Includes information on types of depression, symptoms and where to get help.

Fibromyalgia

Teitelbaum, Jacob. *From Fatigued to Fantastic!* New York, NY: Avery Publishing Group, 2001.

Myers Cocktail. For free referrals to practitioners trained to administer it, contact the American College for Advancement in Medicine at www.acam.org or 23121 Verdugo Dr., Suite 204, Laguna Hills, CA 92653; (888) 439-6891.

Glycemic Index

The Glycemic Index: www.glycemicindex.com. Offers a database of foods with their glycemic measures from the University of Sydney in Australia.

Hormone Replacement Therapy

American College for Advancement in Medicine: www.acam.org. 23121 Verdugo Dr., Suite 204, Laguna Hills, CA 92653; (888) 439-6891. For practitioners trained in natural hormone replacement.

College Pharmacy: www.collegepharmacy.com. Compounding pharmacy specializing in natural, customized HRT therapies; (800) 888-9358.

Life Extension Foundation: www.lef.org/protocols/prtcl-130.shtml. Information on natural hormone replacement for men.

Somers, Suzanne. *The Sexy Years: Discover the Hormone Connection—The Secret to Fabulous Sex, Great Health, and Vitality, for Women and Men,* New York, NY: Three Rivers Press, 2004.

Women's International Pharmacy: www.womensinternational.com. Compounding pharmacy, specializing in natural, customized HRT therapies; (800) 279-5708.

Hypnosis

National Board for Certified Clinical Hypnotherapists: www.natboard.com/index_files/Page548.

htm. 1110 Fidler Lane, Suite 1218, Silver Spring, MD 20910; (301) 608-0123 or (800) 449-8144. Provides a state-by-state database of hypnotherapists.

Intestinal Health

Crook, William G. *The Yeast Connection: A Medical Breakthrough,* New York, NY: Vintage, 1986.

Irritable Bowel Syndrome

Hoffman, Ronald. *Seven Weeks to a Settled Stomach,* New York, NY: Simon and Schuster, 1991.

Mitochondrial Support

NADH/ENADA: www.nadh.com; (800) 928-NADH (6234).

Propax with NT Factor: www.propax.com; (800) 982-9158.

Neurotransmitters

NeuroScience Inc. www.neurorelief.com. Specializes in the assessment and correction of neurotransmitters and hormones. Provides testing, and therapeutic and technical support; (888) 342-7272.

Osteoporosis

Osteosupport. Order at www.drhoffman.com/page.cfm/336 or (800) 456-9384.

Salad and Salmon Diet

Visit: www.drhoffman.com/page.cfm/21.

SAM-e

Brown, Richard and Carol Colman, *Stop Depression Now: SAM-e: The Breakthrough Supplement that Works as Well as Prescription Drugs,* New York, NY: Berkley Trade, 2000.

Stress Reduction

American Institute of Stress: www.stress.org/about.htm. Clearinghouse for stress information

Meditation Internet Resources: www.holisticmed.com/www/meditation.html.

Stress Management and Emotional Wellness Links: http://imt.net/%7Erandolfi/StressLinks.html. Dozens of links to stress management resources from Optimal Health Concepts.

Stress Relief Strategies: www.holisticmed.com/stressfree.html. Good overview of severe stress reduction techniques and resources to learn more.

Transcendental Meditation Program: www.tm.org. Website offers meditation techniques and over 500 studies about the health and brain benefits of meditating.

Syndrome W

Mogul, Harriette R. and Diane Stafford. *Syndrome W: A Woman's Guide to Reversing Mid-Life Weight Gain,* New York, NY: M. Evans and Co., 2005: http://syndromew.com.

Thyroid Function

Armour Thyroid: Available from Forest Pharmaceuticals, Inc. at www.armourthyroid.com or (800) 678-1605, ext.7301.

Shomon, Mary J., *Living Well with Hypothyroidism,* New York, NY: HarperCollins/Harper Resource, 2005.

Thyroid Disease Information Source: www.thyroid-info.com. Provides articles, links, and books for people with thyroid diseases.

Chapter 11: Preparing for Surgery and Recovery

Acidophilus

Lactobacillus GG: www.culturelle.com/index.jsp. Supplements available in most drugstores from Culturelle.

Acupuncture

Auriculotherapy Certification Institute: www.auriculotherapy.org. Online directory of certified ear acupuncture practitioners.

National Certification Commission for Acupuncture and Oriental Medicine: www.nccaom.org/home. htm. 11 Canal Center Plaza, Suite 300, Alexandria, VA 22314; (703) 548-9004. Online directory of practitioners certified in acupuncture, Oriental medicine, Chinese herbology, and Asian bodywork therapy.

Books

Deardorff, William W. and John L. Reeves II. *Preparing for Surgery: A Mind-Body Approach to Enhance Healing and Recovery,* Oakland, CA: New Harbinger Publications, 1997.

Huddleston, Peggy. *Prepare for Surgery, Heal Faster: A Guide of Mind-Body Techniques:* Angel River Press, 2002. Order at www.healfaster.com.

Oz, Mehmet, Ron Arias, and Lisa Oz. *Healing from the Heart: A Leading Heart Surgeon Explores the Power of Complementary Medicine,* New York, NY: E.P. Dutton, 1998.

Bromelain

Nature's Plus: To find a store near you, go to: www.naturesplus.com.

Wobenzym: Supplements available from Naturally Vitamins at www.naturally.com and www.wobenzym.com or by calling (888) 766-4406.

Glutamine

L-Glutamine powder: Available from Jarrow Formulas at www.jarrow.com or by calling (800) 726-0886.

Impact

Available from Novartis Medical Nutrition: www.novartisnutrition.com/us/productDetail?id=973&source=summary.

Integrative/Complementary Surgery

Columbia University Medical Center Integrative Medicine Program. Director: Mehmet Oz, MD: www.columbiasurgery.org/cimp/inpat.html or (800) 227-2762.

Vermont Healing Tools Project. Director: Judith Petry, M.D., P.O. Box 1064, Brattleboro, VT 05301; (802) 254-1250. A pioneer in complementary approaches to surgery, offering resources, support, and education for people with critical or chronic illnesses.

Music Therapy

American Music Therapy Association, Inc.: Contact for qualified music therapists in your area. 8455 Colesville Rd., Suite 1000, Silver Spring, MD 20910. Visit www.musictherapy.org or call (301) 589-3300.

Certification Board for Music Therapists: Only organization to certify music therapists. Contact for therapists in your area. 506 E. Lancaster Ave., Suite 102, Downingtown, PA 19335. Visit www.cbmt.org, or call (800) 765-CBMT (2268) or (610) 269-8900.

Nutrition

Salad and Salmon diet: www.drhoffman.com/page.cfm/21.

Second Opinions

American College of Surgeons. "Should You Seek a Consultation (Second Opinion)": www.facs.org/public_info/operation/consult.html.

Videos

Gentle Visions. Thirty-minute, pre-operative, relaxation videotape by Dr. Judith J. Petry. Order at www.sover.net/~jpetry.

Resources
for Physicians

While every effort has been made to include the most up-to-date information at the time of publication, addresses, telephone numbers, e-mail addresses, and website links are subject to change. For information on specific products, refer to previous section on Resources for Patients.

Articles/Reports

"To Err Is Human: Building a Safer Health System." Report by Committee on Quality of Health Care in America, Institute of Medicine of the National Academies. 2000: www.nap.edu/catalog/9728.html.

Sierpina, Victor S. "Teaching Integratively: How the Next Generation of Doctors Will Practice." *Integrative Cancer Therapies* Vol. 3 No. 3 (2004): pp. 201–207.

Article on immunotoxicology—study of how exposure to environmental chemicals suppresses immune response. Immunosciences Lab, Inc. website: www.immuno-sci-lab.com/2003_cat_page83.

Books/Reference Guides

Blumenthal, Mark, *The ABC Clinical Guide to Herbs,* Austin, TX: American Botanical Council, 2003. Order at www.herbalgram.org/default.asp?c=hcpg.

Ernst, Edzard, *The Desktop Guide to Complementary and Alternative Medicine: An Evidence-Based Approach,* San Diego, CA: Mosby, 2001.

Gaby, Alan R. and Jonathan V. Wright. *Nutritional Therapy in Medical Practice, Reference Manual and Study Guide* (2003 edition), Kent, WA: Wright/Gaby Seminars. www.doctorgaby.com/gaby/index.html.

Kligler, Benjamin and Roberta Lee, *Integrative Medicine: Principles for Practice,* Columbus, OH: McGraw Hill, 2004.

Murcott, Toby. *The Whole Story: Alternative Medicine on Trial?* Palgrave Macmillan, 2005.

PDR for Herbal Medicines. 3rd ed., Montvale, NJ: Thomson Healthcare, 2004.

PDR for Nutritional Supplements. Montvale, NJ: Thomson Healthcare, 2001.

Rakel, David, *Integrative Medicine,* Philadelphia, PA: W.B. Saunders, 2003

Sierpina, Victor, *Integrative Health Care: Complementary and Alternative Therapies for the Whole Person,* Philadelphia, PA: F.A. Davis, 2001.

Courses/Seminars/Professional Training (see also "Professional Organizations Offering Conferences and CME")

American Botanical Council: Provides CME credit for physicians on herbal medicines: www.herbalgram.org or call (800) 373-7105.

Excellence Shock Wave Therapy: www.eswtusa.com. Training and credentialing organization that provides ESWT training to physicians. Includes information on this non-invasive, drugless pain relief treatment for orthopedic conditions.

"Nutritional Therapy in Medical Practice." Course by Alan R. Gaby, M.D., and Jonathan V. Wright, M.D. Wright/Gaby Seminars. Provides state-of-the-art information on the use of diet, nutrients, hormones, herbs, and other natural substances in medical practice: www.doctorgaby.com/gaby/page4.html#Anchor-The-35882.

Drug-Nutrient Interactions

Boullata, Joseph I. and Vincent T. Armenti. *Handbook of Drug-Nutrient Interactions,* Totowa, NJ: Humana Press, 2004.

Center for Food-Drug Interaction Research and Education: www.druginteractioncenter.org. New online tool with section for physicians to check interactions offered by the University of Florida and Tufts University.

Drug-Nutrient Workshop: www.nutritionworkshop.com. User-friendly software for health care professionals to view documented or hypothetical reactions that might occur when conventional drugs are combined with herbs, vitamins and minerals, or other supplements. Applied Nutrition, Inc., 133 East 73 St., Suite 308, New York, NY 10021.

McCabe, Beverly J., Eric H. Frankel, and Jonathan J. Wolfe. *Handbook of Food-Drug Interactions,* Boca Raton, FL: CRC Press, 2003.

Medical Testing Labs

Consumer Lab: www.consumerlab.com. Provides independent test results on hundreds of vitamins, herbs, and natural products to help consumers and doctors evaluate their nutritional content.

Doctor's Data, Inc.: www.doctorsdata.com. An independent reference laboratory providing data on levels of toxic and essential elements in hair, and elements, amino acids, and metabolites in blood and urine. For information on tests and services, call (800) 323-2784.

Genova Diagnostics: www.gdx.net. Offers full range of clinical tests, including for hormonal, allergic, and other conditions. Or information on tests and services, call (800) 522-4762.

Immunosciences Lab, Inc.: www.immuno-sci-lab.com/index2.html. Develops esoteric tests and helps clinicians in the diagnosis of very complex diseases where the immune system is directly or indirectly involved. For information on tests and services, call (800) 950-4686.

Metametrix Clinical Laboratory: www.metametrix.com. Offers a full range of tests, including metabolic profiles, hormone profiles and oxidative stress indicators. For information on tests and services, call (800) 221-4640.

Professional Journals

Alternative Medicine Alert: www.ahcpub.com/ahc_root_html/products/newsletters/ama.html. Monthly newsletter offering busy clinicians evidence-based summaries on alternative and complementary therapies, published by Thomson American Health Consultants.

Alternative Medicine Review: www.thorne.com/index/mod/amr/a/amr. Peer-reviewed studies and research, published by Thorne Research Inc.

Alternative Therapies in Health and Medicine: www.alternative-therapies.com/at/login/index.jsp. Peer-reviewed studies and information on the practical use of alternative therapies in preventing and treating disease.

American Journal of Clinical Nutrition: www.ajcn.org. Published by the American Society for Clinical Nutrition.

Complementary Health Practice Review: www.sagepub.com/journal.aspx?pid=356. Examines topics and trends in practice of CAM.

Focus on Alternative and Complementary Therapies: www.ex.ac.uk/FACT. Review journal of the latest complementary medicine findings.

Holistic Primary Care: News for Health and Healing: www.holisticprimarycare.net. Online and print publication offering scientific information on holistic medicine. Print version reaches 100,000 physicians nationwide.

Journal of Alternative and Complementary Medicine: www.liebertpub.com/publication.aspx?pub_id=26. Peer-reviewed studies and information on therapies outside realm of allopathic medicine.

Journal of the American College of Nutrition: www.jacn.org.

Townsend Letter for Doctors & Patients: www.townsendletter.com. Balanced, scientific information on variety of alternative medicine topics.

Professional Organizations Offering Conferences and CME

American Academy of Anti-Aging Medicine (A4M): www.world-health.net/a4m.html.

American Academy of Environmental Medicine: www.aaem.com. 7701 East Kellogg, Suite 625, Wichita, KS 67207; (316) 684-5500.

American College for Advancement in Medicine: www.acam.org. 23121 Verdugo Dr., Suite 204, Laguna Hills, CA 92653; (800) 532-3688.

American Holistic Medical Association: www.holisticmedicine.org. 12101 Menaul Blvd., NE, Suite C, Albuquerque, NM 87112; (505) 292-7788.

Institute for Functional Medicine: www.functionalmedicine.org. 411 Pt. Fosdick Drive NW, Suite 305. P.O. Box 1697, Gig Harbor, WA 98335; (800) 228-0622.

Web-based Health Information

American Botanical Council: www.herbalgram.org. Provides news, searchable databases and latest scientific research on herbal medicines; (800) 373-7105. CME credit for physicians.

Council for Responsible Nutrition: www.crnusa.org. 1828 L Street, NW, Suite 900, Washington, DC, 20036-5114; (202) 776-7929. Scientific information on vitamin and herbal supplements.

Homocysteine.net.: www.homocysteine.net/pages/homocysteine/1/abouthcy.html. A website for health professionals.

National Center for Complementary and Alternative Medicine: www.nccam.nih.gov/health. A division of the National Institutes of Health. Provides articles and databases; (888) 644-6226.

National Guideline Clearinghouse: wwwguideline.gov. Clinical guidelines for hundreds of conditions.

Natural Medicines Comprehensive Database: www.naturaldatabase.com. Evidence-based, clinical information on natural medicines updated daily; PDA version available. Doctors with websites can link to consumer database to educate patients.

UpToDate: www.uptodate.com. Latest peer-reviewed mainstream treatment guidelines for hundreds of conditions, updated on continuous basis. Section for physicians and patients allows collaboration on treatment plan.

Vitamin D Council: www.cholecalciferol-council.com. Facts, articles and studies on importance of vitamin D.

VitaSearch: www.vitasearch.com. Free literature search by Clinical Pearls on any health topic with weekly research updates.

Notes

Chapter 1

1. Goodwin, James S. and Michael R. Tangum. "Battling Quackery: Attitudes About Micronutrient Supplements in American Academic Medicine." *Archives of Internal Medicine* Vol. 158 (Nov. 9, 1998): pp. 2187–2191.

2. Gaby, Alan R. and Jonathan V. Wright. *Nutritional Therapy in Medical Practice, Reference Manual and Study Guide* (2001 Edition) Kent, WA: Wright/Gaby Seminars; www.doctorgaby.com/gaby/index.html.

3. Fairfield, Kathleen M. and Robert H. Fletcher. "Vitamins for Chronic Disease Prevention in Adults." *Journal of the American Medical Association* Vol. 287, No. 23 (June 19, 2002): pp. 3116–3126.

4. Kuperman, Albert S. "What's Ahead for Med Ed?" *Einstein* (Winter 2004), pp. 12–15.

5. Touger-Decker, Riva. "Nutrition Education of Medical and Dental Students: Innovation Through Curriculum Integration." *American Journal of Clinical Nutrition* Vol. 79, No. 2 (February 2004): pp. 198–203.

6. Cohen, M. and D. Eisenberg. "Potential Malpractice Liability Risk Associated with CAM Therapies." *Annals of Internal Medicine* Vol. 136 (2002): pp. 596–603.

Chapter 2

1. Dr. Lorraine Day's website: www.dr-lorraine-day.com/ (accessed February 14, 2006).

2. Starfield, Barbara. "Is U.S. Health Really the Best in the World?" *Journal of the American Medical Association* Vol. 284, No. 4 (July 26, 2000): pp. 483–485.

3. Dobson, Al, Joan DaVanzo, Maria Consunji, et al. "A Study of the Cost Effects of Daily Multivitamins for Older Adults." The Lewin Group. Presented at *Multivitamins and Public Health: Exploring the Options* meeting, Washington, D.C. (Oct. 1–2, 2003); published January 2004: www.lewin.com/Lewin_Publications/Special_Populations/WyethMultivitaminReport.htm.

4. Rubenstein, Sarah. "Health Plans Embrace Alternatives." *Wall Street Journal* (September 22, 2004): p. D7.

5. Radimer, Kathy, Bernadette Bindewald, Jeffery Hughes, et al. "Dietary Supplement Use by U.S. Adults: Data from the National Health and Nutrition Examination Survey, 1999–2000." *American Journal of Epidemiology* Vol. 160, No. 4 (2004): pp. 339–349.

6. Winslow, Lisa and Howard Shapiro. "Physicians Want Education about Complementary and Alternative Medicine to Enhance Communication with Their Patients." *Archives of Internal Medicine* Vol. 162 (2002): pp. 1176–1181.

7. McGlynn Elizabeth, S.M. Asch, J. Adams, et al. "The Quality of Health Care Delivered to Adults in the United States." *New England Journal of Medicine* Vol. 348, No. 26 (June 26, 2003): pp. 2635–2645.

Chapter 3

1. Hoffman, Ronald. "Mitral Valve Prolapse." *Conscious Choice* (May 1996). http://www.conscious choice.com/holisticmd/hmd093.html.

2. "Doctors' Interpersonal Skills Are Valued More Than Training or Being Up-to-Date." Harris Interactive Poll conducted for the *Wall Street Journal* Online's Health Industry Edition: October 1, 2004. http://www.harrisinteractive.com/news/newsletters/wsjhealthnews/WSJ Online_HI_Health-CarePoll2004vol3_iss19.pdf.

3. Neuman, Fredric, *Worried Sick? The Exaggerated Fear of Physical Illness,* Larchmont, NY: Hadrian Press, 2003.

4. Franklin, Tel. "Part 1: Is Alternative Medicine Really Alternative?" Center for Appreciative Medicine (2003). http://www.appreciativemedicine.com/prof.shtml.

5. "Defining the Patient-Physician Relationship for the 21st Century." Johns Hopkins and American Healthways (Feb. 26, 2004). http://www.patient-physician.com/.

6. Duke Prospective Health Program website. http://www.dukeprospectivehealth.org/ (accessed February 14, 2006).

7. "Complementary and Alternative Medicine in the United States." Committee on the Use of Complementary and Alternative Medicine, Institute of Medicine of the National Academies Board on Health Promotion and Disease Prevention (2005): http://books.nap.edu/catalog/11182.html?onpi_newsdoc01122005.

8. Kindig, David A., Dyanne D. Affonso, and Eric H. Chudler. "Health Literacy: A Prescription to End Confusion." Institute of Medicine of the National Academies (April 8, 2004) http://www.iom.edu/report.asp?id=19723.

9. Beyerstein, Barry L. "Alternative Medicine and Common Errors of Reasoning." *Academic Medicine* Vol. 76 (March 2001): pp. 230–237.

10. People Living with Cancer Live Chat Series: "Complementary and Alternative Medicine and Cancer: What You Should Know" hosted by Dr. Stephen Straus, Director of the National Center for Complementary and Alternative Medicine. http: www.plwc.org/plwc/Main Con structor/1,1744,12-001208-00_14-002003%20Transcripts-00_17-001029-00_18-0030480-00_19-0030482-00_20-001-00_21-008,00.asp (accessed February 14, 2006).

11. Horton, Richard. "The *New* New Public Health Risk and Radical Engagement (editorial)." *Lancet* Vol. 352 (1998): pp. 251–252.

12. Ovamed GmbH website on helminthic therapy: http://www.ovamed.de/english/home/listdaten.php (accessed February 14, 2006).

13. Fox, Barry. "Separating Fact from Fiction: Evaluating Medical Literature." *Journal of the American Nutraceutical Association* Vol. 6, No. 2 (Spring 2003).

14. Moertel C.G., T.R. Fleming, E.T. Creagan, et al. "High-dose Vitamin C Versus Placebo in the Treatment of Patients with Advanced Cancer Who Have Had No Prior Chemotherapy: A Randomized Double-blind Comparison" *New England Journal of Medicine* Vol. 312 (1985): pp. 137–141.

15. Davidson, J.R.T., et al. "Effect of *Hypericum perforatum* (St. John's Wort) in Major Depressive Disorder: A Randomized Controlled Trial." *Journal of the American Medical Association* Vol. 287 (2002): pp. 1807–1814.

16. Whitaker, Julian. "The CAM Sham." *Health and Healing* (October 2004) http://www.dr whitaker.com/c/store_hh_prod2.asp.

Chapter 4

1. Kolata, Gina, "Annual Physical Checkup May Be an Empty Ritual." *New York Times* (August 12, 2003).

2. Sirovich, Brenda E. and H. Gilbert Welch. "Cervical Cancer Screening Among Women Without a Cervix." *Journal of the American Medical Association* Vol. 291 (2004): pp. 2990–2993.

3. Theodosakis, Jason and David T. Feinberg, "When Your Insurance Won't Pay." *Parade* (September 19, 2004).

4. Theodosakis, Jason and David T. Feinberg. *Don't Let Your HMO Kill You: How to Wake Up Your Doctor, Take Control of Your Health, and Make Managed Care Work For You,* New York, NY: Routledge, 2000.

5. Laukkanen, Jari A., Sudhir Kurl, Riitta Salonen, et al. "Systolic Blood Pressure During Recovery From Exercise and the Risk of Acute Myocardial Infarction in Middle-Aged Men." *Hypertension* Vol. 44, No. 6 (December 2004): 820–825.

6. "Body Burden Report." Mount Sinai School of Medicine, Environmental Working Group & Commonweal (January 2003) http://www.ewg.org/reports/bodyburden/es.php.

7. "National Report on Human Exposure to Environmental Chemical" (Reports 1 and 2). Centers for Disease Control and Prevention (March 2001 and January 2003) http://www.cdc. gov/exposurereport/.

8. Siscovick, David S., T.E. Raghunathan, Irena King, et al. "Dietary Intake of Long-Chain n-3 Polyunsaturated Fatty Acids and the Risk of Primary Cardiac Arrest." *Journal of Clinical Nutrition* Vol. 71, No. 1 (January 2000): pp. 208–212.

9. Harris, William S. "Are Omega-3 Fatty Acids the Most Important Nutritional Modulators of Coronary Heart Disease Risk?" *Current Atherosclerosis Reports* Vol. 6 (2004): pp. 447–452.

10. Braly, James and Ron Hoggan. *Dangerous Grains: Why Gluten Cereal Grains May Be Hazardous to Your Health,* New York, NY: Avery Publishing Group, 2002.

Chapter 5

1. Solomon, Caren G., and Robert G. Dluhy. "Bariatric Surgery—Quick Fix or Long-Term Solution?" *New England Journal of Medicine* Vol. 351, No. 26 (December 23, 2004): pp. 2751–2752.

2. Zack, Matthew M., David G. Moriarty, Rosemarie Kobau, et al. "Worsening Trends in Adult

Health-Related Quality of Life and Self-Rated Health—United States, 1993–2001." *Public Health Reports* Vol. 119, No. 5 (2004): pp. 493–505.

3. Marvel, Kim M., R.M. Epstein, K. Flowers, et al. "Soliciting the Patient's Agenda: Have We Improved?" *Journal of the American Medical Association* Vol. 282, No. 10 (September 8, 1999): pp. 942–943.

4. Charon, Rita. "Narrative Medicine." University of Alaska Anchorage, LitSite Alaska website: http://litsite.alaska.edu/healing/medicine.html (accessed February 14, 2006).

5. Boullata, Joseph. "Natural Health Product Interactions with Medications." *Nutrition in Clinical Practice* Vol. 20, No. 1 (February 2005): pp. 33–51.

6. Parker-Pope, Tara. "Why It's Hard to Get a Second Opinion (And How To Make Sure You Get One)." *Wall Street Journal* (February 1, 2005): D1.

Chapter 6

1. Wald, Nicholas J. and Malcolm R. Law. "A Strategy to Reduce Cardiovascular Disease by More Than 80%." *British Medical Journal* Vol. 326 (June 28, 2003): p. 1419.

2. Franco, Oscar H., Luc Bonneux, Chris de Laet, et al. "The Polymeal: A More Natural Safer and Probably Tastier (Than the Polypill) Strategy to Reduce Cardiovascular Disease by More than 75%." *British Medical Journal* Vol. 329 (December 18, 2004): pp. 1447–1450.

3. Harris, William S. "Are Omega-3 Fatty Acids the Most Important Nutritional Modulators of Coronary Heart Disease Risk?" *Current Atherosclerosis Reports* Vol. 6 (2004): pp. 447–452.

4. Kris-Etherton, Penny M., William S. Harris, and Lawrence J. Appel. "AHA Scientific Statement: Fish Consumption, Fish Oil, Omega-3 Fatty Acids, and Cardiovascular Disease." *Circulation* Vol. 106, No. 21 (November 19, 2002): pp. 2747–2757.

5. Fourth International Study of Infarct Survival Collaborative Group. "ISIS-4: A Randomized Factorial Trial Assessing Early Oral Captopril, Oral Mononitrate, and Intravenous Magnesium Sulphate in 58,050 Patients with Suspected Acute Myocardial Infarction." *Lancet* Vol. 345 (1995): pp. 669–685.

6. Schneider, Robert H., C.N. Alexander, F. Staggers, et al. "A Randomized Controlled Trial of Stress Reduction in African Americans Treated for Hypertension for Over One Year." *American Journal of Hypertension* Vol. 18, No. 1 (January 2005): pp. 88–98.

7. Bonaa K.H., I. Njolstad, P.M. Ueland, et al. "Homocysteine Lowering and Cardiovascular Events after Acute Myocardial Infarction." *New England Journal of Medicine* Vol. 354, No. 15 (April 13, 2006): pp. 1578–1588.

8. Lonn E., S. Yusuf, M.J. Arnold, et al. "Homocysteine Lowering with Folic Acid and B Vitamins in Vascular Disease." *New England Journal of Medicine* Vol. 354, No. 15 (April 13, 2006): pp. 1567–1577.

9. Miller, Edgar R., Roberto Pastor-Barriuso, Darshan Dalal, et al. "Meta-Analysis: High Dosage Vitamin E Supplementation May Increase All-Cause Mortality." *Annals of Internal Medicine* Vol. 142 (January 4, 2005): pp. 37–46.

10. Bjelakovic, G., D. Nikolova, R.G. Simonetti, et al. "Antioxidant Supplements for Prevention of Gastrointestinal Cancers: A Systematic Review and Meta-Analysis." *Lancet* Vol. 364, No. 9441 (October 8, 2004): pp. 1219–1228.

11. Boullata, Joseph. "Natural Health Product Interactions with Medication." *Nutrition in Clinical Practice* Vol. 20 (February 2005): pp. 33–51.

12. Cheung, M.C., X.Q. Zhao, A. Chait, et al. "Antioxidant Supplements Block the Response of HDL to Simvastatin-Niacin Therapy in Patients with Coronary Artery Disease and Low HDL." *Arteriosclerosis, Thrombosis and Vascular Biology* Vol. 21 (2001): pp. 1320–1326.

13. Kuller, L.H. "A Time to Stop Prescribing Antioxidant Vitamins to Prevent and Treat Heart Disease?" *Arteriosclerosis, Thrombosis and Vascular Biology* Vol. 21 (2001): p. 1253.

14. Women's Health Initiative. National Heart Lung and Blood Institute: http://www.nhlbi.nih.gov/whi/index.html (accessed February 14, 2006).

15. "Effects of Estrogen or Estrogen/Progestin Regimens on Heart Disease Risk Factors in Postmenopausal Women." The Postmenopausal Estrogen/Progestin Interventions (PEPI) Trial. The Writing Group for the PEPI Trial. *Journal of the American Medical Association* Vol. 273, No. 3 (January 18, 1995): pp. 199–208.

Chapter 7

1. Leaf, Clifton. "Why We're Losing the War on Cancer (and How to Win It)." *Fortune* (March 22, 2004): pp. 77–94.

2. Jo, Jeong-Youn, Elvira Gonzalez de Mejia, and Mary Ann Lila. "Effects of Grape Cell Culture Extracts on Human Topoisomerase II Catalytic Activity and Characterizations of Active Fractions." *Journal of Agricultural and Food Chemistry* Vol. 53, No. 7 (2005): pp. 2489–2498.

3. Takezaki, T., et al. "Dietary Factors and Lung Cancer Risk in Japanese with Special Reference to Fish Consumption and Adenocarcinomas." *British Journal of Cancer* Vol. 84, No. 9 (May 4, 2001): pp. 1199–1206.

4. Clarke, Larry C., Gerald F. Combs, Jr., and Bruce W. Turnbull. "Effects of Selenium Supplementation for Cancer Prevention in Patients with Carcinoma of the Skin: A Randomized Controlled Trial." *Journal of the American Medical Association* Vol. 276, No. 24 (December 25, 1996): pp. 1957–1963.

5. Goodwin, Pamela J., Marguerite Ennis, Kathleen I. Pritchard, et al. "Diet and Breast Cancer: Evidence that Extremes in Diet Are Associated with Poor Survival." *Journal of Clinical Oncology* Vol. 21, No. 13 (July 2003): pp. 2500–2507.

6. Ravasco, Paula, Isabel Monteiro-Grillo, Pedro Marques Vidal, et.al. "Dietary Counseling Improves Patient Outcomes: A Prospective, Randomized, Controlled Trial in Colorectal Cancer Patients Undergoing Radiotherapy." *Journal of Clinical Oncology* Vol. 23, No. 7 (March 1, 2005): pp. 1431–1438.

7. Labriola, Dan. *Complementary Cancer Therapies: Combining Traditional and Alternative Approaches for the Best Possible Outcome,* Roseville, CA: Prima Lifestyles, 2000.

8. Kennedy, Deborah D., Elena J. Ladas, Susan R. Rheingold, et al. "Antioxidant Status Decreases in Children with Acute Lymphoblastic Leukemia During the First Six Months of Chemotherapy Treatment." *Pediatric Blood and Cancer* Vol. 44, No. 4 (April 2005): pp. 378–385.

9. Pathak, Ashutosh K., Manisha Bhutani, Randeep Guleria, et al. "Chemotherapy Alone vs. Chemotherapy Plus High-Dose Multiple Antioxidants in Patients with Advanced Non-Small Cell Lung Cancer." *Journal of the American College of Nutrition* Vol. 24, No. 1 (February 2005): pp. 16–21.

10. Lamson, David and Matthew Brignall. "Antioxidants in Cancer Therapy: Their Actions and Interactions with Oncologic Therapies." *Alternative Medicine Review,* Vols. 4 & 5, Nos. 2 & 5 (1999–2000).

11. "Facts about Cancer Pain Part 2: Non-Drug Treatments for Pain." Supplement to *Alternative Medicine Alert* Vol. 8, No. 3 (March 2005): pp. S1–S4.

12. Padayatti, S.J., H. Sun, Y. Wang, and H.D. Riordan, et al. "Vitamin C Pharmacokinetcs: Implications for Oral and Intravenous USe." *Annals Internal Medicine* Vol. 140 (April 6, 2004): pp. 533–537.

13. Sontag, Susan. *Illness as Metaphor,* New York, NY: Farrar, Straus & Giroux, 1978.

14. Kiecolt-Glaser, Janice K. and Ronald Glaser. "Psychoneuroimmunology and Cancer: Fact or Fiction?" *European Journal of Cancer* Vol. 35, No. 11 (October 1999): pp. 1603–1607.

15. Hansen, Pernille E., Birgitta Floderus, Kirsten Frederiksen, et al. "Personality Traits, Health Behavior, and Risk for Cancer: A Prospective Study of a Swedish Twin Cohort." *Cancer* Vol. 103, No. 5 (March 1, 2005): pp. 1082–1091.

Chapter 8

1. Bjordal, Jan Magnus, Anne Elisabeth Ljunggren, Atle Klovning, et al. "Non-Steroidal Anti-Inflammatory Drugs, including Cyclo-oxygenase-2 Inhibitors, in Osteoarthritic Knee Pain: Meta-Analysis of Randomized Placebo-Controlled Trials." *British Medical Journal* Vol. 329 (December 4, 2004): p. 1317.

2. Neame, Rebecca, A. Hammond, and C. Deighton. "Need for Information and for Involvement in Decision Making among Patients with Rheumatoid Arthritis: A Questionnaire Survey." *Arthritis and Rheumatism* Vol. 53, No. 2 (April 15, 2005): pp. 249–55.

3. Haahr, Jens Peder, S. Østergaard, J. Dalsgaard, et al. "Exercises Versus Arthroscopic Decompression in Patients with Subacromial Impingement: A Randomized, Controlled Study in 90 Cases with a One-Year Follow-up." *Annals of the Rheumatic Diseases* Vol. 64 (2005): pp. 760–764.

4. Sandoval, Manuel, Randi M. Charbonnet, Nataly N. Okuhama, et al. "Cat's Claw Inhibits TNF-alpha Production and Scavenges Free Radicals: Role in Cytoprotection." *Free Radical Biology and Medicine* Vol. 29, No. 1 (July 1, 2000): pp. 71–78.

5. Dial, Elizabeth J., Amanda J. Dohrman, Jim J. Romero, et al. "Recombinant Human Lactoferrin Prevents NSAID-induced Intestinal Bleeding in Rodents." *Journal of Pharmacy and Pharmacology* Vol. 57, No. 1 (2005): pp. 93–97.

6. Holden, Wendy, J. Joseph, and L. Williamson, "Use of Herbal Remedies and Potential Drug Interactions in Rheumatology Outpatients. *Annals of Rheumatic Diseases* Vol. 64 (2005): p. 790.

7. Schanberg, Laura E., Karen M. Gil, Kelly K. Anthony, et al. "Pain, Stiffness, and Fatigue in Juvenile Polyarticular Arthritis: Contemporaneous Stressful Events and Mood as Predictors." *Arthritis & Rheumatism* Vol. 52, No. 4 (April 7, 2005): pp. 1196–1204.

8. Trentham, David E., "Oral Tolerization as a Treatment of Rheumatoid Arthritis," *Rheumatic Disease Clinics of North America* Vol. 24 (1998): pp. 525–536.

9. "Diet and Your Arthritis: A Look at the Research." Arthritis Foundation: http://www.arthritis.org/resources/nutrition/diet.asp (accessed February 14, 2006).

10. Trollmo, C., M. Verdrengh, and A. Tarkowski. "Fasting Enhances Mucosal Antigen Specific B cell Responses in Rheumatoid Arthritis." *Annals of Rheumatic Diseases* Vol. 56 (February 1997): pp. 130–134.

11. Kjeldsen-Kragh, J. "Mediterranean Diet Intervention in Rheumatoid Arthritis," *Annals of Rheumatic Diseases* Vol 62 (March 2003): pp. 193–195.

12. Dunlop, Dorothy D., Pamela Semanik, Jing Song, et al. "Risk Factors for Functional Decline in Older Adults with Arthritis." *Arthritis & Rheumatism* Vol. 52, No. 4 (April 2005): pp. 1274–1282.

13. Bates, Betsy. "Using Yoga to Ease OA Pain." *Family Practice News* Vol. 34, No. 21 (November 1, 2004): p. 49.

14. Harlow, Tim, Colin Greaves, Adrian White, et al. "Randomised Controlled Trial of Magnetic Bracelets for Relieving Pain in Osteoarthritis of the Hip and Knee." *British Medical Journal* Vol. 329 (December 18–25, 2004): pp. 1450–1454.

15. Walsh, Nancy. "Acupuncture Improves Knee OA in Phase III Study." *Family Practice News* Vol. 35 No. 2 (January 15, 2005): p. 55.

16. Hadjivassiliou, M., D.S. Sanders, R. A. Grünewald, et al, "Gluten Sensitivity Masquerading as Systemic Lupus Erythematosus." *Annals of Rheumatic Diseases* Vol. 63 (2004): pp. 1501–1503.

17. Straub, R.H. and Cutolo M. "Involvement of the Hypothalamic-Pituitary-Adrenal/Gonadal axis and the Peripheral Nervous System in Rheumatoid Arthritis. Viewpoint Based on a Systemic Pathogenetic Role." *Arthritis and Rheumatism* Vol. 44, No. 3 (2001): pp. 493–507.

Chapter 9

1. Boeve, Bradley. J. McCormick, G. Smith, et al. "Mild Cognitive Impairment in the Oldest Old." *Neurology* Vol. 60 (2003): pp. 477–480.

2. Sheline, Yvette I., Milan Sanghavi, Mark A. Mintun, et al. "Depression Duration but Not Age Predicts Hippocampal Volume Loss in Medically Healthy Women with Recurrent Major Depression." *The Journal of Neuroscience* Vol. 19, No. 12 (June 15, 1999): pp. 5034–5043.

3. Galanis, Daniel J., C. Joseph, K.H. Masaki, et al. "A Longitudinal Study of Drinking and Cognitive Performance in Elderly Japanese-American Men: the Honolulu-Asia Aging Study." *American Journal of Public Health* Vol. 90, No. 8 (August 2000): p. 1254.

4. Podewils, Laura J., Eliseo Guallar, Lewis H. Kuller, et al. "Physical Activity, APOE Genotype, and Dementia Risk: Findings from the Cardiovascular Health Cognition Study." *American Journal of Epidemiology* Vol. 161, No. 7 (2005): pp. 639–651.

5. Elias, Penelope K., Merrill F. Elias, Michael A. Robbins, et al. "Blood Pressure-Related Cognitive Decline: Does Age Make a Difference?" *Hypertension* Vol. 44 (2004): pp. 631–636.

6. Kaplan, R., E. Greenwood, G. Winocur, et al. "Dietary Protein, Carbohydrate, and Fat Enhance Memory Performance in the Healthy Elderly." *American Journal of Clinical Nutrition* Vol. 74 (2001): pp. 687–693.

7. Yaffe, Kristine, Alka Kanaya, Karla Lindquist, et al. "The Metabolic Syndrome, Inflammation, and Risk of Cognitive Decline." *Journal of the American Medical Association* Vol. 292, No. 18 (November 10, 2004): pp. 2237–2242.

8. de la Monte, Suzanne M. and Jack R. Wands. "Review of Insulin and Insulin-like Growth Factor Expression, Signaling, and Malfunction in the Central Nervous System: Relevance to Alzheimer's Disease." *Journal of Alzheimer's Disease* Vol. 7 (2005): pp. 63–80.

9. Lian, Xiao-Yuan, Zhizhen Zhang, and Janet L. Stringer. "Protective Effects of Ginseng Components in a Rodent Model of Neurodegeneration." *Annals of Neurology* Vol. 57, No. 5 (April 25, 2005): pp. 642–648.

10. Yang, Fusheng, Giselle P. Lim, Aynun N. Begum, et al. "Curcumin Inhibits Formation of Amyloid Oligomers and Fibrils, Binds Plaques, and Reduces Amyloid in Vivo." *Journal of Biological Chemistry* Vol. 280, No. 7 (February 18, 2005): pp. 5892–5901.

11. Addolorato, Giovanni, D. Di Giuda, G. De Rossi, et al. "Regional Cerebral Hypoperfusion in Patients with Celiac Disease." *American Journal of Medicine* Vol. 116, No. 5 (March 1, 2004): pp. 312–317.

Chapter 10

1. Heath, Iona. "Who Needs Health Care—the Well or the Sick?" *British Medical Journal* Vol. 330 (April 23, 2005): pp. 954–956.

2. Kravitz, Richard L., Ronald M. Epstein, and Mitchell D. Feldman. "Influence of Patients' Requests for Direct-to-Consumer Advertised Antidepressants." *Journal of the American Medical Association* Vol. 293, No. 16 (April 27, 2005): pp. 1995–2002.

3. Alpert, Jonathan E., D. Mischoulon, and G.E.F. Rubenstein. "Folinic Acid (Leucovorin) as an Adjunctive Treatment for SSRI-Refractory Depression." *Annals of Clinical Psychiatry* Vol. 14, No. 1 (March 2002): pp. 33–38.

4. Coppen, A. and J. Bailey. "Enhancement of the Antidepressant Action of Fluoxetine by Folic Acid: A Randomized, Placebo-Controlled Trial." *Journal of Affective Disorders* Vol. 60 (November 2000): pp. 121–30.

5. Shanahan, Fergus and Peter J. Whorwell. "IgG-Mediated Food Intolerance in Irritable Bowel Syndrome: A Real Phenomenon or an Epiphenomenon?" *American Journal of Gastroenterology* Vol. 100, No. 7 (July 2005): pp. 1558–1559.

Chapter 11

1. Hensrud, D.D., D.D. Engle, and S.M. Scheitel. "Underreporting the Use of Dietary Supplements and Nonprescription Medications among Patients Undergoing a Periodic Health Examination." *Mayo Clinic Proceedings* Vol. 74 (1999): pp. 443–447.

2. Ang-Lee, Michael K., Jonathan Moss, and Chun-Su Yuan. "Herbal Medicines and Perioperative Care." *Journal of the American Medical Association* Vol. 286, No. 2 (July 11, 2001): pp. 208–216.

3. Cook, J.W., L.M. Pierson, W.G. Herbert, et al. "The Influence of Patient Strength, Aerobic Capacity and Body Composition upon Outcomes After Coronary Artery Bypass Grafting." *The Thoracic and Cardiovascular Surgeon* Vol. 49, No. 2 (April 2001): pp. 89–93.

4. Broadbent, Elizabeth, Keith J. Petrie, Patrick G. Alley, et al. "Psychological Stress Impairs Early Wound Repair Following Surgery." *Psychosomatic Medicine* Vol. 65, No. 5 (September/October 2003): pp. 865–869.

5. Petry, Judith, J. "Surgery and Complementary Therapies: A Review." *Alternative Therapies in Health and Medicine* Vol. 6, No. 5 (September 2000): pp. 64–76.

6. Barrera, Rafael, Weiji Shi, David Amar, et al. "Smoking and Timing of Cessation: Impact on Pulmonary Complications After Thoracotomy." *Chest* Vol. 127 (June 2005): pp. 1977–1983.

7. Petry, Judith, J. "The Body as Battlefield." LearningPlaceOnline.com. (1998): http://www.learningplaceonline.com/illness/choices/body-battlefield.htm (accessed February 14, 2006).

8. Delgado-Rodríguez, M., M. Mariscal-Ortiz, A. Gómez-Ortega, et.al. "Alcohol Consumption and the Risk of Nosocomial Infection in General Surgery." *British Journal of Surgery* Vol. 90, No. 10 (October 2003): pp. 1287–1293.

9. Braga, Marco, Luca Gianotti, Andrea Vignali, et al. "Preoperative Oral Arginine and N-3 fatty Acid Supplementation Improves the Immunometabolic Host Response and Outcome After Colorectal Resection for Cancer." *Surgery* Vol. 132 (2002): pp. 805–814.

10. Nathens, Avery B., Margaret J. Neff, Gregory J. Jurkovich, et al. "Randomized, Prospective Trial of Antioxidant Supplementation in Critically Ill Surgical Patients." *Annals of Surgery* Vol. 236, No. 6 (December 2002): pp. 814–822.

11. Faure, Henri, et al. "Zinc in Surgery." *The Journal of Nutritional Medicine* Vol. 3 (1992): pp. 129–136.

12. Gan, Tong J., Kui Ran Jiao, Michael Zenn, et al. "A Randomized, Controlled Comparison of Electro-Acupoint Stimulation or Ondansetron Versus Placebo for the Prevention of Postoperative Nausea and Vomiting." *Anesthesia & Analgesia* Vol. 99 (2004): pp. 1070–1075.

13. Wang, Shu-Ming, Carol Peloquin, and Zeev N. Kain. "The Use of Auricular Acupuncture to Reduce Preoperative Anxiety." *Anesthesia and Analgesia* Vol. 93 (2001): pp. 1178–1180.

14. Calò, Leonardo, Leopoldo Bianconi, Furio Colivicchi, et al. "N-3 Fatty Acids for the Prevention of Atrial Fibrillation After Coronary Artery Bypass Surgery: A Randomized, Controlled Trial." *Journal of the American College of Cardiology* Vol. 45 (May 17, 2005): pp. 1723–1728.

15. Tepaske, R., H.T. Velthuis, H.M. Oudemans-van Straaten, et al. "Effect of Preoperative Oral Immune-Enhancing Nutritional Supplement on Patients at High Risk of Infection after Cardiac Surgery: A Randomised Placebo-Controlled Trial." *Lancet* Vol. 358 (2001): pp. 696–701.

Conclusion

1. Fadiman, Anne. *The Spirit Catches You and You Fall Down: A Hmong Child, Her American Doctors, and the Collision of Two Cultures,* New York, NY: Farrar, Straus & Giroux, 1997.

2. Garrow, Donald and Leonard E. Egede. "Association Between Complementary and Alternative Medicine Use, Preventive Care Practices, and Use of Conventional Medical Services Among Adults with Diabetes." *Diabetes Care* Vol. 29, No. 1 (January 2006): pp. 15–19.

Index